POWERED BY ADHD

POWERED BY

ADHD

Strategies and Exercises
for Women to Harness
Their Untapped Gifts

AMELIA KELLEY, PhD

ZEITGEIST • NEW YORK

All rights reserved.
Published in the United States by Zeitgeist™,
an imprint and division of Penguin Random House LLC, New York.
zeitgeistpublishing.com

Zeitgeist™ is a trademark of Penguin Random House LLC.
ISBN: 9780593690031
Ebook ISBN: 9780593886465

Cover design by Katy Brown
Interior design by Erin Yeung
Cover and interior art © Shutterstock/Olga Rai
Author photograph © by Jeannene Matthews, JR Photography 2023
Edited by Kim Suarez

Printed in the United States of America
1st Printing

To all the women

diagnosed with ADHD,

those who have coped in silence,

and the people who love

and support them.

CONTENTS

Introduction

Nearly eight million American adults have attention-deficit/hyperactivity disorder (ADHD). However, many women do not receive proper diagnosis until their late thirties to early forties. Once diagnosed, women can encounter a great deal of confusion about how to navigate symptoms and, on the flip side, fully realize the gifts of having ADHD. As a mental health clinician with over 20 years of experience working with neurodiversity—specifically individuals with ADHD and highly sensitive people (HSPs)—I have dedicated my career to helping these people realize their full potential to achieve fulfilling, successful, and joy-filled lives.

In addition to my professional work, both my family history of neurodiversity as well as my own, and being married to someone with ADHD, have taught me the many strengths and abilities of ADHD that often go unrecognized. This lack of recognition is further compounded by gender disparity in research, despite the fact that ADHD occurs as frequently in women as it does in men. Society's lack of awareness about women with ADHD and how they fit into the world often negatively affects how they live their lives. One might see a woman with ADHD and mistake her energy for overexuberance or being manic, or perhaps her hyperfocus on a task comes off as inattention to other pressing matters. When others misunderstand the gifts that women with ADHD offer, this can lead to feelings of inferiority, fear, and shame. Further issues involve society's expectations that young girls and women ought to be more agreeable and compliant, which leads to harmful effects such as masking symptoms and prolonging proper diagnosis and support.

My mission is to highlight the enormous strengths, talents, and skills that go hand-in-hand with ADHD, especially for those who work to learn helpful skills and use tools to empower themselves. And that's where this book comes in. *Powered by ADHD* guides this transformative experience by harnessing your unique strengths and gifts, while exploring the potential issues that occur when ADHD isn't understood or managed properly. This book has been curated to be highly practical, flexible, and focused on self-compassion—a combination that can produce immediate results and improve everyday life. Perhaps most importantly, this book will encourage you not to conform to neurotypical ideals or hide your abilities, but to embrace who you truly are. Gifted. Strong. And ready to learn. Let's go!

How to Use This Book

Let curiosity and self-compassion lead the way in reading this book. As you do, *Powered by ADHD* will offer knowledge, clear up misunderstandings, and shed light on what you may have overlooked about ADHD. It'll provide a greater understanding of your remarkable brain and how it interacts with the world around you.

Chapter 1 explores how ADHD affects women and challenges outdated beliefs about ADHD. Because we are constantly learning more about neurodiversity and the ADHD brain, this chapter offers a breadth of information about current research and attitudes. You'll also get the chance to take an ADHD self-assessment, which you can present to your healthcare provider for their review and assessment.

In chapter 2, we'll discuss how living as a woman with ADHD can cause challenges that aggravate false notions about the diagnosis. You'll also begin to see how previously held beliefs may have been holding you back and causing what's known as "ADHD trauma."

Through stories, Chapters 3 through 6 will examine the unique strengths that women with ADHD possess. Since there is no "one-size-fits-all" when describing women with ADHD, examples of clients and women with ADHD shared in this book will reflect nuances about the different challenges each face, and the skills that help overcome them.

The second part of the book—chapters 7 through 12—will explore various areas in women's lives: work or school, home, finances, parenting, self-care, and relationships. Within each area, you'll find research-supported solutions that can help you use your gifts in practical, everyday ways. For a holistic perspective, it's recommended to read each chapter in its entirety, getting a comprehensive look at the different areas that ADHD impacts.

As you read, mark the challenges you struggle with. Then revisit the strategies provided so you can practice applying these skills long-term. Most of us fall out of sync with coping skills from time to time. If this happens, try not to get discouraged—just return to what you know works for you. The stories, skills, and knowledge you gain from this book will help you rethink ADHD—from an issue to overcome, to a set of adaptive traits with its own gifts—that when harnessed effectively, richly enhance you and the world around you.

PART I

EMBRACING THE ADHD BRAIN

WE'RE ABOUT TO CHALLENGE what has been previously taught about ADHD being a disorder and reframe it as an evolutionary adaptation that offers unique skills and strengths (that can also be challenging at times) for women with the diagnosis or women with strong ADHD traits. Instead of seeing ADHD simply as a "deficit" or "disorder," we will learn why the ADHD brain differs from the "typical" brain and consider how women with ADHD add tremendous value to society—a gift that only grows when they are given the strategies to harness their skills.

Chapter One

Rethinking ADHD

This chapter explores how ADHD has been understood by the clinical community to date, and the ways it impacts women and girls in today's society. Common coping strategies don't always align with the strengths of the ADHD brain, and this chapter uses the latest research to paint a new outlook that is much brighter and full of potential than ever before for women with the diagnosis.

Women and ADHD

Nobody has to tell you that being a woman can be difficult in today's world! Juggling professional and personal commitments, navigating relationships, bumping up against societal walls, ceilings, and stereotypes, and trying to excel at the countless roles we take on can become overwhelming—for a woman with ADHD, it can be that much harder.

Attention-deficit/hyperactivity disorder (ADHD) is a medical diagnosis involving neurodevelopmental issues in the ability to focus. Contrary to popular belief, those with ADHD do not *lack* focus or attention; rather, they have issues with regulating their focus and shifting their attention away from things they find interesting or engaging. The result is a myriad of symptoms that can occur to some degree (depending on the person) and disrupt everyday life, including:

- Impulsivity

- Disorganization

- Trouble prioritizing

- Poor time management

- Difficulty staying attentive (depending on the task)

- Trouble multitasking

- Restlessness

- Poor planning

- Tendency toward frustration

- Stress coping issues

- Mood swings

- Irritability

Many of these symptoms manifest from trying to fit into a world designed for the non-ADHD brain—that is, a world that requires sustained attention and inactivity in highly controlled settings. As technology shifts our world toward endless stimulation and demanding, hyper-structured educational and professional settings as the societal norm, it's perhaps unsurprising that the diagnosis of ADHD is rising. In fact, it is reductive to say that ADHD has become "more common," since the demands placed on women to multitask (Supermom, anyone?) have increased symptom presentation. Another driving factor behind this trend is a generally heightened awareness, sometimes even sparked by the diagnosis of their children.

While ADHD is increasingly being diagnosed in women, this diagnosis still lacks the early detection and intervention found in regard to boys and men. Writer and TEDx keynote speaker Martha Barnard-Rae revealed that, up until the late 1990s, all ADHD research was conducted on males, and it was not until 2002 that the first study piloted to explore its impact on women was conducted. Here's one reason: the disruptive and impulsive traits of ADHD found in many boys and men appear less commonly in young girls and women with ADHD, making it more difficult for educators and family members to detect.

There is still much to learn about ADHD in women, but a few symptoms of ADHD shown to be common to women include:

- Increased anxiety

- Feelings of restlessness

- Feeling mentally "on the go"

- Feeling overwhelmed in social situations

In 1997, an analysis of research on gender differences in ADHD showed that, among girls, the diagnosis commonly goes undetected by teachers because, as previously mentioned, girls tend to act out less than their male counterparts. The results also show that these same girls faced more exclusion from their peers, leading to greater difficulties than boys in areas of social and educational development.

While awareness of ADHD in girls and women has grown since the 1990s, it's not yet where it should be. Sufficient ongoing research is necessary to further reduce stigma and support the lives of women with ADHD.

ADHD Self-Assessment

If you suspect you have symptoms of ADHD, it can be helpful to complete the following ADHD self-assessment, based on the *Diagnostic and Statistical Manual of Mental Disorders* and tailored specifically to women. Your results can serve as a starting point to share with your healthcare provider, who can offer a proper diagnosis. After each question, check the box that applies most closely to you.

1. Do you feel as if life is out of control and it's impossible to meet demands?
   — Very Often   — Rarely
   — Often   — Never
   — Sometimes

2. Do you watch others of equal intelligence and education pass you by in achievement?
   — Very Often   — Rarely
   — Often   — Never
   — Sometimes

3. Do you start the day determined to get organized, and end the day feeling defeated?
   — Very Often   — Rarely
   — Often   — Never
   — Sometimes

4. Is your time and energy taken up with coping, staying organized, finding lost items and holding it together, with seemingly no time for fun or relaxation?
   — Very Often   — Rarely
   — Often   — Never
   — Sometimes

5. Do you hesitate to have people over to your home because you're ashamed of the mess?

— Very Often   — Rarely

— Often   — Never

— Sometimes

6. Does time, money, clutter, or "stuff" dominate your life and hamper your ability to achieve your goals?

— Very Often   — Rarely

— Often   — Never

— Sometimes

7. Does it seem like you waver between feeling like either a "couch potato" or a "tornado of energy"?

— Very Often   — Rarely

— Often   — Never

— Sometimes

8. Do you have difficulty concentrating in social situations, even when someone is speaking directly to you?

— Very Often   — Rarely

— Often   — Never

— Sometimes

9. Do requests for "one more thing" at the end of the day put you over-the-top emotionally?

— Very Often   — Rarely

— Often   — Never

— Sometimes

10. Do you feel physically uncomfortable when you need to remain still?

— Very Often   — Rarely
— Often   — Never
— Sometimes

11. Is it difficult for you to shut out sounds and distractions that don't seem to bother others?

— Very Often   — Rarely
— Often   — Never
— Sometimes

12. How often do you have difficulty unwinding and relaxing when you have time to yourself?

— Very Often   — Rarely
— Often   — Never
— Sometimes

13. When in conversation, how often do you find yourself finishing other people's sentences?

— Very Often   — Rarely
— Often   — Never
— Sometimes

14. Do you feel like others lead consistent, regular lives while you struggle?

— Very Often   — Rarely
— Often   — Never
— Sometimes

15. Do you despair about fulfilling your potential and meeting your goals?

— Very Often   — Rarely

— Often   — Never

— Sometimes

16. Do you feel like you are passing for "normal," but you are really masking other thoughts, feelings, or behaviors?

— Very Often   — Rarely

— Often   — Never

— Sometimes

17. Do you feel overwhelmed in busy places (like stores, the office, school, or at parties)?

— Very Often   — Rarely

— Often   — Never

— Sometimes

18. How often do you leave things to the last minute?

— Very Often   — Rarely

— Often   — Never

— Sometimes

NOTE: This self-test is not intended to diagnose or replace the care of a healthcare professional. Only a doctor or mental health professional can diagnose ADHD based on clinical evaluation. If you scored "Very Often" or "Often" on at least half of the items in this check list, you may want to explore the potential of having ADHD.

A World Not Designed for ADHD

For someone with ADHD, the world would be a much better place if, instead of viewing ADHD as a medical disorder, it was viewed as a form of diversity. The term "neurodiverse" is used to describe anyone whose brain develops and works differently than the average neurotypical person. Neurotypical does not mean correct or better; it simply refers to the majority of those who do not have the clinical symptoms present in divergences such as ADHD.

Neurodivergences can run the gamut. In the book *Unmasking Autism: The Power of Embracing our Hidden Neurodiversity,* psychologist Devon Price purports that neurodiversity includes any person in a state of extreme stress or imbalance. In addition to ADHD, this could include eating disorders, trauma, learning disabilities, sensory processing sensitivity, autism, schizophrenia, mood disorders, and others. In fact, most of us can become neurodivergent under certain circumstances; it's only that there are varying levels, with some divergences being genetic and congenital in nature.

Despite most people having some degree of divergence, it still seems we are trying to conform to a narrow box of "normal." This is especially true of what we expect of children and adults with ADHD. But what if the world was designed equally for those with ADHD and those without? Up until the last century, this seemed to be the case. Those with skills and traits that helped humanity also possessed evolutionary traits aligned with aspects of ADHD. These people were hunters, voyagers, military personnel, farmers, and factory workers, and they became the leaders and backbone of our country.

Today, however, we find ourselves in the thick of change. Industries are evolving rapidly due to smart automation, and many lucrative jobs involve formalized development training, 40-hour work weeks, and the previously discussed "sustained attention and inactivity in highly controlled settings." These types of jobs don't always support the way the more experiential and creative ways the ADHD brain learns and excels.

EXECUTIVE FUNCTIONS IMPAIRED BY STRESS

FOR ALL WOMEN (WITH AND WITHOUT ADHD)

Difficulty sustaining attention	Working memory deficits	Distraction and forgetfulness
Problems with self-control	Trouble starting tasks and transitioning between activities	Inability to multitask or plan
Issues with emotion regulation	Difficulty managing time when on task	Trouble following conversations and remembering names

ADDITIONALLY, FOR WOMEN WITH ADHD

Trouble listening when spoken to	Tendency to interrupt often and talk excessively
Excessive fidgeting	Hyperfocusing if passionate about a subject

Meanwhile, jobs that capitalize on the gifts and skills of those with ADHD are generally compensated at a lower rate. In this way, today's society is favoring one way of thinking over the other, causing an imbalanced hierarchy, and impacting socioeconomic class, ideas around success, and the confidence and self-esteem of those who don't conform to the formally structured workplace mindset.

If ADHD Came with a Manual

Supporting women with ADHD means fully understanding how they learn and how their learning impacts their executive functions. Executive functions are mental skills that include working memory, flexible thinking, and self-control. Stress can impact the effectiveness of these skills. In fact, according to psychologist Thomas Brown, anyone can struggle with these skills when under stress, leading to a variety of challenges. For those with ADHD, the list grows even longer.

According to Russell Barkley, an ADHD pioneer, executive functioning is not a product of environment or upbringing; rather, it is a product of genetics. What this means is that for women with ADHD, executive functioning is primarily affected by neurological activity related to the way their brain works as opposed to life stress. Any issues with executive functioning aren't character flaws—they are simply part of a person's DNA, and there are ways to cope with them. Studies show similar impairments in executive functioning between genders, and many of the common executive functioning strategies such as making lists, calendar planning, or just simply "trying to stay focused" seem to fail for both men and women with ADHD. Still, there are specific executive functioning challenges women with ADHD experience related to societal norms and social pressures placed on women, such as:

- Multitasking
- Planning far ahead, especially for families and social events

- Being social without being withdrawn
- Having self-control and not seeming too "loud," "aggressive," or "hyperactive"

These skills often conflict with the natural wiring of the ADHD brain. For example, in social settings, many women with ADHD require a little space (withdrawing) to process everything going on around them.

"The Holistic Psychologist," Nicole LePera, took to social media to challenge the messaging around women being able to "do it all." She highlighted how this harmful messaging has conditioned women to over-function, often single-handedly juggling a career, parenting, caring for extended family, and running a home. The belief that a woman must forfeit their well-being for others is dangerous messaging that can cause exhaustion, mental illness, and burnout. For women with ADHD who already struggle with executive functioning, this expectation is even more damaging, rendering it nearly impossible to engage in proper self-care, manage their diagnosis, and expand on the gifts ADHD has to offer.

What women and all individuals with ADHD deserve is the truth: the truth about how our brains function, what unique challenges ADHD can pose to executive functioning, what strengths to draw from, and what coping skills will and won't work. Essentially, what we need is a proper manual offering an entirely new outlook on ADHD that empowers us to understand our experiences and quiet the expectations and pressures that come from a neurotypical world. Thankfully, research continues, and we can educate ourselves through resources such as healthcare providers, support groups and organizations, and books like the one you're reading.

Part of any healing process involves acknowledging our struggles. Silence is the antecedent to shame, while awareness and expression allow for growth and learning new ways to become self-empowered. When ADHD goes unidentified and untreated, it can damage self-perception and mental health, leading to complex forms of trauma, which will be explored in the next chapter.

Chapter Two

ADHD Trauma and Coping Solutions

Difficulties that come up in living with ADHD, whether diagnosed or not, can create pain and trauma for adult women. Trauma is not always one harrowing event—it can also be a series of distressing experiences, making it difficult to function. Healing from trauma takes time and energy, which can divert resources away from managing ADHD symptoms. For a woman to fully embrace their strengths, it is important to understand what kind of trauma they may be dealing with, if any. From there, they can confront these traumas and develop appropriate coping solutions, helping them to realize their strengths and gifts as a woman with ADHD.

Shame

According to famed researcher Brené Brown, shame is an "intensely painful feeling or experience of believing that we are flawed and therefore unworthy of love and belonging."

I was working with a client with ADHD on a goal she had set. As she processed her shame around not meeting her goal, she began to feel restless. She said she wanted to jump out of her skin and began to sob into her lap. As I comforted her, she expressed how ashamed she was of her fidgeting, because she used to get in trouble in school for doing it, which led to her parents grounding her for weeks on end. She shared that even now, as an adult, she was constantly worried about what others thought of her when she couldn't sit still—at work, with her friends, and especially when with her family. She had never spoken about this to anyone because she was ashamed and self-conscious. She was even worried what I, her therapist, would think of her. Her internal belief that she was flawed was so strong that it made receiving love and support difficult, even when it was offered to her. I assured her that sharing her story took courage, and whether she knew it or not, it was a first step toward healing.

Coping Solution: Share Your Shame

Shame differs from guilt. Both make us feel bad, but guilt relates to feeling responsible for a perceived or real harmful behavior or attitude, and often leads us to action (such as leaving a note on a car if you dinged it). Guilt is about what you did or didn't do, not who you believe you are. Shame is the internalized belief or personification about who you are, derived from harmful feelings about oneself. While guilt leads to corrective action, shame thrives from inaction. Therefore, when we speak about our shame, its intensity begins to dissipate. Sharing our shame opens us up to authentic connection and allows others to support us.

Answer the following prompts to address potential shame you are experiencing.

1. To help cope with shame, identify one person who you feel safe with. This could be someone who shares their own shame stories and knows how to actively listen without shutting your feelings down.

    _____

    _____

2. Now take a moment to reflect on something related to your ADHD that you have experienced shame around. Be compassionate and gentle with yourself. Try to choose only one thing to start, and write it below.

    _____

    _____

    _____

3. Next, imagine what it would feel like to share what you wrote with this person. Identify any feelings and sensations that come up for you and recognize your physical symptoms of shame.

    _____

    _____

    _____

    _____

4. Finally, when you are ready, share what you wrote. Consider how it made you feel. If it feels good to do so, you can share more.

5. Remind yourself often that you are not your shame; rather, your shame is a mental and emotional pressure created from holding in your stories.

When we are the only one hearing the plot of our internal dialogue, we tend to favor the negative. Sharing your thoughts and feelings with a safe person can pull you out of a shame spiral and lead you back toward self-compassion.

Rejection Sensitivity

Because ADHD poses many challenges with executive functioning, those with ADHD face hurdles and mishaps beginning at an early age. This, combined with unhelpful ableist messaging, misunderstanding, judgment, and disability-related discrimination, leads them to experience an intense emotional response to criticism or rejection. This stands to reason; one study shows that, in school alone, a child with ADHD could receive 20,000 corrective or negative comments by the time they are 10. It's therefore understandable that this form of ADHD trauma holds people back from trying new things or taking on challenges they fear they may not succeed at. I see many highly gifted and skilled clients with ADHD afraid to take healthy risks, which further affirms the unhelpful belief that if and when they face rejection, they won't be able to cope. They manifest the very thing they fear—failure—by never trying.

Coping Solution: Practice Failing

What is one of the most effective ways to overcome rejection sensitivity? Practice failing. In the viral TED Talk, "What I learned from 100 days of rejection," entrepreneur Jia Jiang shared his radical approach to overcoming rejection sensitivity by purposely trying to be rejected for 100 consecutive days. Many people did reject him, but to his surprise, some said yes to even the most off-the-wall requests (such as asking employees at Krispy Kreme to turn his donuts into the shape of the Olympic rings). The payoff in the end? Surviving rejection and understanding that he could tolerate it.

Practice this skill by trying the following:

1. Think of something you've been uncertain about trying (starting a new hobby, applying for a job, asking out a love interest).
2. Set a day and time you will go for it.
3. Detach from the outcome and see success as the effort only, not the result.
4. Aim to fail daily (read on to learn why).

Most people who accomplish amazing things fail countless times before they succeed. The story of Thomas Edison (who displayed ADHD symptoms) is a famous example of an individual experiencing multiple failures before hitting ultimate success—he failed thousands of attempts before finally succeeding at inventing the first lightbulb.

When mastering failure:

• Pay attention to stories you may tell yourself (if they are shame stories, share them!) and sensations you experience in your body.

• If you notice tension when taking risks or attempting challenging things, try methods to relax into the discomfort such as breath work or other grounding techniques.

• Try to sustain a compassionate growth mindset, where you focus on what you're learning from your mistakes instead of chastising yourself for making them. You are bravely stepping out there—be proud!

Masking

Driven by shame around the diagnosis, many women with ADHD believe they should present themselves as neurotypical and will go through exhaustive efforts to hide their neurodiversity. Some examples of ADHD masking include:

- Repressing what you want to say by not speaking up or speaking quietly

- Constantly checking your belongings to ensure you haven't lost anything

- Mirroring others' social cues and reactions instead of behaving naturally

- Suppressing stimming behaviors and fidgeting by doing something "socially acceptable" like bouncing your leg

- Developing perfectionistic tendencies as a result of the anxiety around making mistakes

ADHD researcher and neuropsychologist Russell Barkley coined the term "impression management" to describe these masking behaviors, and states that this camouflaging of symptoms occurs in at least one-third of adults with ADHD. One might suspect that, in women, who are highly socialized to adjust to other's needs, masking would be even more present.

Many issues occur as a result of masking ADHD, including delayed diagnosis and treatment. The effort it takes to constantly mask ADHD can also lead to anxiety, depression, low self-esteem, substance abuse, and other forms of ADHD trauma. Until the world becomes more tolerant of neurodiversity, and ADHD is not seen as something people feel they need to conceal, there are some helpful ways to cope.

Coping Solution: Choose Your Masks Wisely

Some masking skills can be helpful, such as repressing the desire to run around the room during a meeting, or triple-checking where you put your keys. Conversely, some masking behaviors are unnecessary and potentially harmful to your sense of self. Complete the following prompts to understand your own masking behaviors.

List a few ways you mask that you find helpful.

1. _____

2. _____

3. _____

Now, consider masking skills that you feel are more repressive of your personality, such as not laughing loud at jokes, or digging your nails into your thighs to keep yourself from fidgeting.

List a few ways you mask that you find repressive.

1. _____

2. _____

3. _____

Now, find someone else who either has ADHD or considers themselves neurodiverse (or has empathy for those who are). Check in with them about what masking behaviors they use, compare them to your own. You may find that your shame around these behaviors doesn't align with their actual severity (remember my client who was so concerned with her fidgeting—after sitting all day, I'm sure I was fidgeting just as much as she was). Sometimes the ideas behind masking are simply not accurate, and choosing instead to celebrate your unique self will bring more joy than the feeling of blending in.

Ruptured Relationships

Relationship trauma stems from a history of negative emotional or physical experiences with somebody a person cared about or who played an important role in their life. Not everyone with ADHD has experienced relationship trauma, but this form of trauma is prevalent for those with

ADHD for many reasons. Many people with ADHD encounter difficulty in relationships because of rejection sensitivity or insecurities. Somebody might not understand why their friend isn't always listening, forgets important dates, or interrupts them frequently, and as a result, they might end the relationship or distance themselves without knowing why these things were happening. This kind of abandonment can result in trust issues, causing those with ADHD to believe that everyone is against them.

Many of the single women with ADHD who I work with in my practice have trouble dating because they fear being abandoned. This can result in an insecure attachment style, leading to other relationship problems. Finding a healthy relationship requires them to unmask their symptoms and express their genuine selves to the person they're dating, including their diagnosis and even any associated shame. This level of authenticity is no small task for someone trying to heal after numerous failed or ruptured relationships.

Coping Solution: Practice a Secure Attachment Pattern

The way we react in relationships, especially when we fear conflict or abandonment, is indicative of our attachment style. Based on the theory developed by researchers John Bowlby and Mary Ainsworth, there are four primary attachment styles: anxious, avoidant, disorganized, and secure. For the sake of coping with relationship trauma from ADHD, we'll focus on how to practice the healthiest form: secure attachment.

The good news is that attachment style is very flexible and can be adjusted based on the relationships you are in and efforts you put forth. To work toward secure attachment and cope with feelings of mistrust in others, focus on the following:

- Identify and distance yourself from those in your life who are not securely attached.

- Continue learning about your attachment style so you can identify when you are reacting from a wounded space as opposed to a secure space. An excellent book on this topic is *Anxiously Attached: Becoming More Secure in Life and Love* by couples counselor Jessica Baum.

- Journal your reactions and emotions about relationships. Go back and reflect when not in a reactive state.

- Actively communicate your wants and needs. This will always lead you toward your secure parts.

SECURE ATTACHMENT INVOLVES THE ABILITY TO:

- Regulate emotions

- Trust others

- Communicate wants and needs

- Seek emotional support

- Manage interpersonal conflict

- Forgive

- Reflect on relationships

- Be alone

- Connect with others

- Be emotionally accessible

It takes time to establish a new attachment style, so be patient and compassionate with yourself. Having supportive people around you can help rewire your brain to feel comfortable with close connections.

Finding Strength

When considering how to make the world better and brighter for people with ADHD, we must redefine the diagnosis as being an adaptive trait with an abundance of useful strengths and gifts. As you work to repair ADHD trauma, you will likely discover unique skills and strengths within yourself that may have been previously overlooked.

A necessary step in overcoming any ADHD trauma is learning to embody the diagnosis. This means accepting the differences in the ADHD brain that can cause challenges, but also the parts that are gifts. In the following chapters, we will dive into some of these strengths and explore how each strength translates into a particular skill set. We will also explore how to manage and maximize these strengths, helping you retain control over other areas of your life.

Chapter Three

The Gift of Creativity

The following chapter explores the ADHD gift of creativity and how it manifests as a unique set of skills and advantages. With creativity being the root of discovery and innovation, women with ADHD have the potential to become pioneers in all of life's ventures.

Powered by Creativity

Creativity means having the ability to generate ideas and alternatives and solve problems in unique ways. It's often associated with the ADHD brain because this form of neurodiversity has an enhanced ability to use imagery while problem-solving. Often described as a "wandering mind," the creative ADHD brain comes up with novel and unusual ideas simply by interacting with the world in different ways than those without ADHD.

At its foundation, creativity includes curating unique ideas as well as effectively communicating these ideas or solutions to others. In this way, women with ADHD cannot only "think outside the box," but according to researcher Tara Chaplin, they are also shown to possess greater emotional expressivity than their neurotypical peers, in relation to both positive emotions and internalized sadness. By recognizing and harnessing the creative skills enhanced by ADHD, women can build confidence and leverage these skills to spark impactful ideas, innovations, and solutions.

Untapped Gifts

Women with ADHD often possess the following skills:

Innovation. Women with ADHD are excellent at forming new ideas due to their heightened ability to use a skill called **divergent thinking**, which is the ability to think of many ideas from one single starting point. Examples of divergent tasks include being inventive and finding new ways to use everyday objects. To enhance this skill, give yourself the time and space needed to remember and organize these creative thoughts when they come up. Perhaps keep a journal on hand to jot down ideas. This will give you a reference to reflect from and share as you wish.

Broadened imagination. One of the qualities that makes women with ADHD creative is their openness to ambiguity. They push boundaries of norms such as generalized rules, ideas, expectations, and even how something should look or appear. This form of imagination broadening is called **conceptual expansion**, and those with ADHD outperform their neurotypical counterparts in this ability. An example from the research includes asking participants, both with and without ADHD, to create something new (such as drawing a novel animal that does not exist on earth). Those with ADHD created more novel and imaginative animals than those without ADHD, who were more likely to reference previously held knowledge of an animal. This is an example of **knowledge constraint**, which is more common with the non-ADHD brain.

Curiosity. Women with ADHD often get distracted when something is interesting, even if their attention should be elsewhere. This unconscious shift in focus is not due to a lack of discipline; rather it is a form of heightened curiosity referred to as "Zetetic thinking style." This style of thinking and attention occurs when someone becomes easily curious or engaged in new ideas and interests, even if there is a cost associated with inquiry (for example, being distracted during an important meeting at work by beautiful flowers outside the window, which leads to a curiosity about horticulture, which leads to planning a future flower bed). While the stream of curiosity can become problematic when it precludes other responsibilities, when applied to creativity, this passion and excitement can lead to innovative ideas.

Successful Women with the ADHD Gift of Creativity

Countless women with ADHD have shared their gifts of creativity with the world, and if we are lucky, many more will continue to do so.

When people think of ADHD, many tend to picture a person who can't sit still or concentrate—someone perhaps with a short attention span. It may interest you to learn about Greta Gerwig. She is an actress, writer, and director, who has written and directed films such as *Lady Bird*, *Little Women*, and *Barbie*. She is also a woman with ADHD. As a child, Gerwig was said to have an abundance of energy, another ADHD gift. But it's her filmmaking creativity that has dazzled audiences. Gerwig is proof that the sky's the limit for a creative woman with ADHD.

Strengthening Your Creativity

Environments such as school and work can present difficulties for women with ADHD; however, environments that support creativity allow their gifts to flourish.

Self-compassion is an integral part of encouraging creativity. Instead of thinking of the ADHD mind as being "distractible" or "chaotic," we can take a more helpful and accurate perspective of "curious, innovative, and imaginative." If you are a woman with ADHD with a penchant for creativity:

- Surround yourself with people and opportunities that encourage your gift.

- Choose to focus less on limiting expectations around ADHD; let the sky be the limit.

- Accept mistakes as an essential part of the creative process.

Doing any of the above will strengthen your natural gift of creativity enhanced by the ADHD brain. It will also encourage what's called a **growth mindset**, which further enhances the ability to create and will be explored more extensively later in this book.

Chapter Four

The Gift of Hyperfocus

This chapter will explore the ADHD gift of hyperfocus and how it manifests as a unique set of skills and advantages in women's lives. Hyperfocus is unique to the ADHD brain, as it's the contrary ability to effectively focus on a mass scale. Women with ADHD who harness their ability to hyperfocus find mastery in task completion and intensified dedication to a skill, craft, or task. When harnessed, it is truly a superpower. But like with any superpower, it is important to know what to do when hyperfocus become problematic.

Powered by Hyperfocus

Hyperfocus is an extraordinary gift of ADHD that looks like long periods of time fully absorbed in something that's fun or interesting to the exclusion of everything else. According to research, hyperfocus is more present in those with ADHD than those without. When thinking about ADHD, many imagine someone with a short attention span who struggles to focus in general; a more accurate description would be that those with ADHD struggle to regulate where their attention goes.

The field of positive psychology describes hyperfocus as "flow," or a state of intense concentration on the present moment. Many describe it as feeling "in the zone." Some benefits of this include:

• Time passing more quickly on a task

• Increased confidence and "can-do" attitude

• Reduced self-consciousness

• Feelings of joy and satisfaction

Hyperfocus is a state many people try to attain. However, it's easy to see how this kind of tunnel vision might interfere with other areas of life. Picture researching something you find exciting. Here, the tradeoff may be missing out on sleep or being late to important engagements due to being overly immersed in the research. To take full advantage of this gift, it's important to bolster the positive skills involved with hyperfocus while setting effective boundaries with time, energy, and triggers for such selective focus.

Untapped Gifts

Productivity. Poor task completion is often considered a symptom of ADHD; however, this doesn't paint the entire picture. In hyperfocus, those with ADHD can achieve unimaginable goals and deadlines under time pressure! A client I work with once expressed her confidence in knocking out a task last minute because it's "what she does," and she does it well. While this can sometimes be seen as procrastination, it can also be quite effective if managed in the right way.

Individuals with ADHD perform more effectively at tasks with clearly defined goals and more immediate deadlines—creating pressure that increases the stimulation demanded of that task. The result is an increased release of the chemical messenger dopamine, which further enhances attention toward achieving a goal as well as positive feelings about oneself.

To ensure that the skills of hyperfocus enhance task completion, it's important to consider how much time you truly need to accomplish a task, while still allowing for a shorter, time-focused approach. Stretching a task out over days can lead to boredom and avoidance. Instead, you can set mini deadlines for yourself—this approach offers dopamine rewards delivered by task completion at a more regular rate, and helps you stay on track and aware of time.

Managers and co-workers of those with ADHD often find them to be the best people to approach with a tight deadline or exciting project, as long as they are provided with clear time limits and milestones. Giving someone with ADHD an open-ended time goal does not tap into their ability to hyperfocus and makes becoming distracted more likely.

Mastery. Ever heard of the 100-hour rule? The idea is that if you spend 18 minutes a day on a task or goal, by the end of one year you will have spent at least 100 hours mastering something, making you better than 95 percent of the rest of the world at any given discipline. Impressive, sure, but if you add the ADHD superpower of hyperfocus, your time commitment to an interest can easily become 200 or 300 hours by the end of a year. Many individuals who are referred to as savants are often not born that way; rather, they possess the ability to hyperfocus on a task. Consider one of the most famous intellects of our time, Albert Einstein. As intelligent and focused as he was on mathematics and science, many say his personality was equally disorganized and spontaneous. If you move aside and allow a woman with ADHD to put as much energy as they want into something they care about, they can surpass all expectations.

Refinery. Another characteristic of hyperfocus includes the more positive aspects of perfectionism (without the negative self-criticism). When applied directly to perfecting a skill, the ADHD brain operates with elevated attention, causing everything unrelated to diminish. If a woman with ADHD is interested in something, they are more likely to refine that skill than their non-ADHD counterparts, simply because they will be drawn to invest more time.

Successful Women with the ADHD Gift of Hyperfocus

Olympic athletes must embody the ability to hyperfocus, as the dedication and focus needed to become a world champion is monumental. One such athlete, who has become a role model for the ADHD community, is gymnast Simone Biles. She has won an astounding 37 Olympic and World Championship medals combined, as well as the Presidential Medal of Freedom. When hackers leaked her medical records, confirming her diagnosis of ADHD, Biles responded with authentic transparency about her diagnosis and the fact that she carries no shame over it. She has credited her gift of hyperfocus in large part for her success at the sport she loves.

Making Hyperfocus Work to Your Advantage

Your environment plays a key role in whether the gift of hyperfocus will benefit you. Specifically, this involves removing things in your space (both physical and virtual) that distract you from accomplishing tasks. Consider your computer screen. You may have a job to do on that computer, but the dopamine rush offered by distractions such as social media can lead to hyperfocusing on the wrong task—the old "rabbit hole" that steals your time. Remedy this by keeping the spaces around you clear of anything unrelated to what you want to accomplish.

Time is another important factor to consider. When you're in a state of hyperfocus, time can pass at astonishing rates. For some, this can become problematic because losing track of time leads to neglecting other priorities and even self-care. A *Time* article, "Playing Tetris Will Make You Forget You're Hungry," cited studies done on game players in the state of hyperfocus and found that they were prone to ignoring physical cues such as sleepiness, hunger, and thirst. One effective way to combat the time warp that hyperfocus can cause is to use the **Pomodoro Technique**: set a length of time for focused work (for example, 25 minutes) followed by a pre-determined break (such as five minutes). Research shows this method increases productivity during the working periods and improves the ability to better track and manage time.

Downtime plays an important role in balancing lengthy states of hyperfocus. During intense states of concentration, the brain can fatigue, leading to stress and increased ADHD symptoms such as irritability, mood swings, and restlessness. Taking time to decompress allows you to process everything you learned or accomplished. It also restores your energy for other executive functions. Reconnecting with other personal needs such as rest and relationships helps create balance with the ADHD gift of hyperfocus, ensuring it remains a superpower.

Chapter Five

The Gift of Energy

Harnessing the gift of energy goes hand-in-hand with getting rest to keep everything in balance. When you achieve this balance, you can engage fully in your experiences with vitality and excitement.

Powered by Energy

Many women who have ADHD feel like they are "always on the go." For some, this translates to feelings of restlessness, but this energy can also be channeled into amazing talents and abilities. This excess energy is due to the ADHD brain thriving when experiencing optimal stimulation. Studies done on students playing with a fidget cube found that the movement helped improve their focus, illustrating how stimulation can help someone with ADHD excel in whatever they are setting their mind to. On his podcast, *The Huberman Lab,* Stanford professor and neuroscientist Dr. Andrew Huberman shared that the ADHD brain functions best when stimulated because it helps to normalize communication between the brain's default mode network (regions of the brain that are active when introspective, such as mind-wandering) and task positive network (regions of the brain that are active when attending to a task). With ADHD, it is important to support harmonious firing of these networks, as opposed to the typical state in which they are both constantly working, but separately.

Stimulant medications can orchestrate these two networks by calming the nervous system and relieving the need to constantly seek stimulation. When ADHD goes unmanaged, the need for stimulation often presents as excess physical energy, commonly seen in young boys. With young girls, it can also present as internalized energy manifesting as anxiety or racing thoughts. When there is nowhere to express this excess energy, it can lead to increased anxiety and internalized shame around the diagnosis. But when a girl or woman has the chance to use a skill that can channel her energy in a positive way, it effectively helps her thrive with the diagnosis.

Untapped Gifts

Physical or athletic advantage. As mentioned, people with ADHD need more stimulation to feel engaged and alert. In some ways, this looks like hyperactivity, but it can also look a lot like athleticism, which means those with ADHD have the potential to excel in sports as well as other physical activities or jobs that demand increased energy.

Research has shown a connection between the energy derived from impulsivity and enhanced athletic performance. There is also evidence that sports that demand quick movements and reactivity, such as baseball and basketball, are well suited for athletes who also have ADHD.

The positive feedback the brain and body receive from engaging in a beloved sport further drives the gift of hyperfocus and improves performance. Beyond sports, when someone with ADHD is physically active, they can improve executive functioning and reduce ADHD symptoms. In this way, the gift of energy can serve as both a coping mechanism and specialized skill.

Passion for relationships. Another gift of energy that exists for those with ADHD is a passion for meaningful connections with others. While ADHD can lend itself to certain social difficulties that we will explore in chapter 12, it can also manifest as a magnetic personality. A study that explored positive aspects of ADHD from the perspective of successful adults discovered that when people with ADHD are feeling their best, they possess exceptional social intelligence, humor, self-acceptance, and recognition of feelings in others. Essentially, when someone with ADHD is provided a supportive space to be themselves, many tend to feel they are "on fire" and fully engaged when meeting new people.

The dopamine reward provided by novel experiences when around new people can become an asset when dating if ADHD is being managed. A desire to connect with a potential love interest can make it easier for someone with ADHD to move past the early awkward stages of getting to know someone and forge toward deeper connection.

Personally, I remember meeting my now-husband (who has since been diagnosed with ADHD) and finding him incredibly engaging, romantic, and attentive. His enthusiasm made it easier for me to open up and connect with him.

The energy someone with ADHD embodies when socializing is not just about the thrill of novelty, but also because they tend to be affected by a phenomenon called **emotional contagion**. Emotional contagion describes the experience of observing someone else's emotions, behaviors, and energy and unconsciously mimicking them. For this reason, it's especially important to protect your energy and emotional state by surrounding yourself with positive, supportive people.

Successful Women with the ADHD Gift of Energy

When considering the gift of energy, actress Cameron Diaz seems to embody this gift in her work and persona. Her bubbly personality practically leaps off the screen, causing viewers to smile right along with her. Once quoted as dropping out of high school after being bullied for her ADHD, Diaz has since channeled her innate qualities and ADHD traits into various positive manifestations, including being one of the highest paid actresses in Hollywood. She has explained that her drive for learning and immersing herself in preparation for acting roles as being attributed to her ADHD. Diaz also published two health books, including *The New York Times* bestseller, *The Body Book: Feed, Move, Understand and Love Your Amazing Body.*

Embracing the Gift of Energy

A common gift of ADHD-related energy is having the passion to leap from challenge to challenge that life presents. But when women with ADHD who crave challenges are not given space to express themselves creatively, mentally, or socially, it can negatively impact their well-being. This kind of repressed energy can lead to substance use, anxiety disorders, insomnia, and chronic pain from inflammation, most commonly in the form of autoimmune disorders. That is why it's so important to prioritize activity and release of energy in whatever way feels right to you.

In addition to saying yes to your passions, it is also important to practice saying "no." Your ADHD energy may inspire you to say yes to every opportunity, but check in with yourself first to make sure you have the resources and energy to follow through. Sometimes a spontaneous idea will lead you to picture the end result without considering the steps needed to get there. Finding a balance between overcoming boredom but not becoming oversaturated takes self-reflection.

For some women, issues with exhaustion or lacking motivation can arise when ADHD is not managed. This can result from inattentive symptoms, or more frequently, a sense of learned helplessness and pervasive expectations of failing. To manage your energy effectively and stave off unhealthy mindsets, ensure that you:

- Get adequate sleep
- Take breaks when hyperfocusing
- Avoid overcommitting to work
- Recognize any increases in anxiety
- Take prescribed medications or supplements as recommended
- Ask for help when needed

Chapter Six

The Gift of Spontaneity

The tendency to act on a whim is a trait of ADHD. But when someone can harness their impulsivity by jumping into life at full force, it becomes the ADHD gift of spontaneity.

Powered by Spontaneity

Spontaneity is central to many of the decisions that release the mind from the status quo and allows other ADHD gifts to manifest. Executing *creative* ideas, with *energy* and passion, leads to *hyperfocus* that allows for mastery. All of these ADHD gifts need a catalyst: a *spontaneous* moment in the mind of someone with ADHD that inspires them to act.

In her famous TED Talk, "How to stop screwing yourself over," motivational speaker Mel Robbins suggests this strategy to harness the spark of spontaneity: start potentially unpleasant tasks within five seconds of thinking about or planning to do them. Robbins, who has ADHD, suggests that it bypasses overthinking, avoidance, and potential anxiety around meeting your goals.

While we all can be spontaneous at times, spontaneity for those with ADHD appears much more natural and unconstrained. When given the chance, women with ADHD seem to burst through the mundane and dive right into their mission. A variety of skills come from this gift—skills that can be tempered by self-compassion and boundaries when necessary.

Untapped Gifts

Risk-taking. Not knowing whether taking chances will work out often leads cautious-minded individuals to refrain from trying, while others make bold choices that can lead to amazing experiences and discoveries. The dopamine reward driven by risk-taking makes it incredibly appealing to some women with ADHD, and the more skilled someone becomes at risk-taking, the more often they will engage in these pursuits.

Look at the world of business, evolving and diversifying with every new day. Today, there are 13 million women-owned businesses in the United States, running the gamut from a home-based shop selling crafts on Etsy to the billion-dollar dating site, Bumble. For a woman with ADHD who likes to take risks, entrepreneurship scratches that itch, satisfying their craving for adventure. And as more women begin running the world of business (currently, women run 10.4 percent of Fortune 500 companies, according to *Fortune* magazine), the list of neurodiverse women taking risks in business will surely grow.

Diversity of talent. As Stephen Tonti shared in his winning TEDx Talk, he is a self-professed director, writer, actor, drummer, scuba diver, soccer player, camera operator, airbrush artist, physicist, star gazer, rock climber, snow boarder, model maker, stage manager, camp counselor, DJ, club president, magician, and, for a brief moment in time, a watch repair man. He then clarified, for anyone wondering, that he also has ADHD. The talk, titled "ADHD as a difference in cognition, not a disorder," explored how the gift of limitless enthusiasm to try new things can result in a multitude of talents, abilities, and positive impacts on the world around us.

He explored how, when given the right support and encouragement, people with ADHD can use their spontaneity in incredible ways. Considering that ADHD does not mean the inability to focus, but rather the difficulty to focus unless something interests you, it would make sense that the more things someone with ADHD tries, the more likely they will remain excited by having the chance to flip focus when desired. For example, if a woman with ADHD develops many interests and skills, she can trick her brain into remaining engaged by changing course and refocusing on something else she enjoys. As she continues to explore, she will continue to find new pursuits that sustain her drive.

Adaptability. Part of trying new things and taking risks includes coming up against barriers and failings. Saying "yes" means trying things that may or may not work out. If they're willing to meet failure in stride, those with ADHD will be much more likely to discover what they truly love. This journey can be difficult, whether it be finding the right partner, job, or life purpose, or managing ADHD symptoms. It's not uncommon for someone with ADHD to take longer to finish school or find the "right" job or direction in life than others, but, during the journey, they are continuously adapting to new situations. This perseverance and persistence are crucial qualities that people with ADHD develop as they grow.

Take, for instance, a typical grade-school classroom in America. By the time children reach sixth grade, they no longer get physical breaks or time to play unless they do sports. Swiftly changing bodies, brains, and hormones equate to dysregulated nervous systems—and for those with ADHD, this is even more difficult to manage. Consequently, children will find ways to cope or receive help in coping. Fidget toys, IEPs, frequent bathroom breaks, tutors, medication, supplements, diet changes—it can take a lot to fit the mold of expectations. Children with ADHD are in a constant state of adapting to environments that are not always designed for them. When someone with ADHD realizes their innate ability to adapt, it can improve self-esteem and facilitate a growth mindset as opposed to a failure schema—creating self-awareness that will serve them well throughout life.

Successful Women with the ADHD Gift of Spontaneity

Lisa Ling, award-winning TV journalist and author, shared that her ADHD was a large contributor to her successful media career. Although she struggled in school as a young girl, she was also given the opportunity to take a risk on something she felt passionate about: journalism. At just 16 years old, she was cast on *Scratch*, a syndicated TV news magazine for teens. Since then, she has reported on *ABC News,* PBS, and *The View*, and has been a correspondent for *The Oprah Winfrey Show* and had her own documentary series, *Our America with Lisa Ling.* She has shared that taking focus breaks and exercising helps channel her impulsive energy into more focused drive for her passion, which has taken her on adventures around the world. As Ling has shown, learning to adapt the gift of spontaneity in a focused way can lead to big rewards.

Being in Charge of Spontaneity

Without spontaneity, many of life's greatest adventures and joys would never be discovered. Being drawn to the unknown and the excitement of novelty is one of the many gifts of ADHD. While this gift can be rewarding, it requires boundaries and focus to flourish. The more anyone, not just those with ADHD, puts on their plate, the more there is to manage. In my practice with ADHD clients, I call this the "cart before the horse syndrome," where ideas flow freely, but the follow-through on the initial spark doesn't always last. It's important to use effective organizational skills to manage passion projects as well as contemplation about how to handle results after making spontaneous choices. For example, you might quit a job and decide to go back to school without forethought or planning. While the choice may be the right one, it can become difficult to manage mundane things like scheduling, finances, and follow-through, because the mundane is where the ADHD brain often loses its spark of spontaneity.

As we move forward, we'll continue to explore practical ways to ensure the gift of spontaneity propels you to take risks, learn new things, and thrive, even when things don't go as planned. Unlearning inaccurate failure schemas and leading with confidence allows women with ADHD to celebrate their spontaneity when given the opportunity to take chances.

PART II

POWERED
BY ADHD

PART II WILL EXPLORE how you can use ADHD strengths to overcome common issues associated with the diagnosis. As you read each scenario, be mindful of your reactions to anything that triggers strong feelings. Honor your needs as you learn the skills, and manage your mental load by revisiting chapter 2 if needed. Many women with ADHD have learned to overlook overwhelming feelings to mask their diagnosis, but tending to your needs can alleviate ADHD symptoms and impart a sense of self-empowerment.

The exercises encourage exploration—this exploration facilitates change. You may also encounter ideas or approaches you've tried before. If you feel any resistance, remember that, with optimism and self-compassion, you'll experience substantial, lasting positive impacts.

Before beginning the strategies and exercises in this book:

- Take a deep breath in, and exhale.
- Find a grounded, calm, and soft space in your body.
- Close your eyes if you wish.
- Lead with curiosity, love, and acceptance.

Chapter Seven

Work

Have you ever felt like you have so much potential that you haven't lived up to? Or know that you could excel if only your boss, professor, or family knew how to support you? Work of any kind—whether on the job, in school or the community, or at home—has a significant impact on our sense of life satisfaction. This chapter explores how to adapt your unique gifts and traits so whatever work you want to do is possible.

FINDING THE RIGHT CAREER

There is no job a woman with ADHD can't do. That said, there are jobs that are more well-suited to your unique gifts and traits. Finding work that fulfills your sense of purpose *and* works well with your ADHD traits takes some consideration. Jobs that tend to suit women with ADHD offer enough challenge, the potential for hands-on work, creative thinking, innovation, variety, physical activity, and the ability to think outside the box. These include writers, editors, entrepreneurs, artists, therapists, librarians, sales reps, ER nurses, first responders, detectives, inventors, educators, and executives, to name a few.

Despite these strengths, women were historically stereotyped and taught from a young age to pursue more traditional jobs, but this has not always served women with ADHD in professional arenas. Thankfully, these dynamics are shifting, and today, women with ADHD might test out a variety of jobs in quest of "the one." For many, finding meaning through work is an integral part of life satisfaction as well as a pipeline to overcoming certain ADHD traumas such as shame or fear of failure.

Finding Your Path

WHAT YOU WILL LEARN

- How to connect with what brings you joy and consider how this can be woven into your work
- How to practice introspection, imagination, and planning

WHAT YOU WILL NEED (IN ADDITION TO TIME)

- A writing utensil
- This book or a journal

ADHD STRENGTH
CREATIVITY

Traditional career assessments are not typically designed for those with ADHD, as they don't account for potential struggles experienced in non-ADHD-friendly work environments—nor do they specify the many strengths unique to ADHD. The following career assessment is created specifically to assist women with ADHD in exploring career options that inspire them and fit with their unique set of skills and needs.

Instructions

Answer the following questions, and then think creatively about how you can integrate what excites you into potential career choices.

1. What are three things that bring me joy? *(If you are interested in something, your ability to hyper-focus and succeed will be more likely.)*

_____

_____

_____

_____

2. What do I most enjoy doing with my time that creates a sense of flow? (*This question explores which ideas and jobs may encourage your gift of hyperfocus.*)

_____

_____

_____

_____

3. Do I prefer working with others or alone? (*It's helpful to determine if you are prone to either distraction from saturation of stimuli, or restlessness when not engaged socially.*)

_____

_____

_____

_____

4. What skills come easily for me, or others have said I am good at? (*This step allows you to work through previous failure schemas and remind you of what you are skilled at.*)

_____

_____

_____

_____

5. What is my ideal work schedule? *(This step accounts for personal preferences, family responsibilities, and sleep difficulties, which we will explore in chapter 11).*

_____

_____

_____

_____

6. What sorts of people do I most enjoy being around? (*Because emotional contagion (page 47) is prevalent in ADHD, it's good to choose a field with people whose traits you would like to emulate*).

_____

_____

_____

_____

For example, as an art therapist who owns my own practice, I might answer the questions like this:

- I enjoy helping people, learning new things, and drawing.

- Spending time with others.

- I prefer working with others, but not large groups.

- I am creative and a good listener.

- I like flexibility in my schedule.

- I like to be around open-minded people.

Finally, using your answers, brainstorm and write out a possible description of your ideal job. If you realize that it aligns with a particular job or field, write that down too.

_____

_____

_____

_____

If you're not sure how your preferences might fit into a career:

- Do an internet search with key words (for example: jobs that are flexible, creative, and autonomous).

- Run your list by a trusted friend or advisor.

- Re-read your list of preferences over the next few days and weeks and see what sticks out as most important to you.

By exploring your answers in this way, you'll identify qualities in your ideal job without being overwhelmed by endless possibilities. This creative approach to exploring your potential career path provides concrete ways to think about your work, which helps the ADHD mind focus.

TIME MANAGEMENT

Time management can be one of the most frustrating challenges for women with ADHD. Recent research has found that time blindness is a potential symptom of ADHD, resulting in procrastinating, delaying work, or missing deadlines entirely. Time blindness can also cause difficulty in accurate time perception when trying to accomplish a task, leading to anxiety around timing and deadlines for work or school. Time blindness can take on many forms, including:

- Losing track of time because of distractions

- Feeling like you don't have a good "internal clock"

- Poor time management

- Impulsivity

- Boredom

- Losing track of time during transitions

- Procrastination

Strength-Based Time Management Plan

By removing barriers created by neurotypical time management, women with ADHD can choose skills that work well for them. If a plan does not work one day, approach yourself with compassion and remain curious about why you struggled. Psychiatrist David Streem created a helpful acronym for checking in on yourself called H.A.L.T. Ask yourself, *Am I Hungry, Angry, Lonely, Tired?* to gain insight as to why you may be struggling with a goal. Then attend to your needs before revisiting your goal.

Instructions

Read over the following strategies for effectively managing time with ADHD as well as some of the barriers that may get in the way of success. Then complete the prompts that follow to guide you in creating your strength-based time management plan.

Eliminate to-do lists. If there is anything you take away from this section, it is to stop using to-do lists. Yes, you may need a list for groceries or when planning an event, but for the most part, the ADHD brain does not thrive well with traditional list-making. To-do lists can be overwhelming for those with ADHD, as there is no limit to what can be added, and prioritizing these tasks can be difficult.

Use a calendar instead—for everything. Calendars are different than to-do lists because they are time-sensitive, and having a certain level of time pressure

WHAT YOU WILL LEARN

- How to use an empowering time management skill to overcome time blindness and manage your time

WHAT YOU WILL NEED (IN ADDITION TO TIME)

- A calendar (virtual or paper)
- A writing utensil (if using a paper calendar)

ADHD STRENGTH HYPERFOCUS

is helpful for those with ADHD when prioritizing their time. To apply this skill:

- Throw out your lists and schedule everything: buying a birthday card, setting up a doctor's appointment, working out, unpacking—all of it. Anything that requires your time goes on the calendar. (If it is difficult to choose a time to do something, you can add it to the day as a "task" which is a feature available in most virtual calendars.)

- Use just one calendar, and always keep it accessible. Some find using their phone easiest; others enjoy hand-writing their tasks in a daily planner.

- If you skip it, reschedule it. Don't ignore it or let it go.

Set up visible cues. Because those with ADHD function best with concrete forms of information, visual cues are essential for managing time. These can include:

- That calendar. Keep it handy and check it often.

- Clocks—arrange them so they are visible in all rooms. You can also get a 60-minute visual countdown timer.

- Concrete reminders. If you know you have to feed the dog in an hour, leave the bowl where you'll see it (or better yet get an automatic feeder like we have in my house!).

Set alarms. Alarms are one of the most effective cues for time management and ADHD. Apply this strategy anytime you need to track time, such as to signal upcoming meetings or to let you know when a break is over, or when you need to leave for class or pick up your kids from school.

Break down tasks. Breaking up tasks into more achievable goals can increase motivation and improve time management. Create a mental map of what needs to be done and set multiple deadlines before the final one. Take, for example, packing to move out of a home:

- Instead of spending all day packing, choose one item to pack (say, picture frames).

- When that is completed, take a break. Even a short break can still be rewarding. Grab a glass of water or check in with a friend or family member about what you accomplished.

- Begin with a new item.

These little successes increase the release of dopamine and reinforce a growth mindset as opposed to a failure schema. Crossing off a task in your calendar can be rewarding and motivating. These moments are also an excellent time to reward yourself with self-care.

MY STRENGTH-BASED TIME MANAGEMENT PLAN

Taking what you learned in the previous section, set your intentions for managing your time going forward.

Ways I struggle most with time management include:

_____

_____

_____

_____

_____

Times I am best able to manage time include:

_____

_____

_____

_____

I will use the following skills from the previous section in my plan:

_____

_____

_____

_____

I will track time using this type of calendar or planner:

_____

_____

_____

_____

Visual cues I can use include:

_____

_____

_____

_____

I will know I have improved with this goal when:

_____

_____

_____

_____

Something I would like to accomplish with my improved time management includes:

_____

_____

_____

_____

A mantra or phrase I will say to encourage myself is:

_____

_____

_____

_____

WORKING FROM HOME

According to the US Census Bureau, the number of Americans working from home tripled from 2019 to 2021 due to the COVID pandemic. Many have returned to the office; however, the influx of work from home jobs is still prevalent. While working from home offers flexibility and relief from potential office distractions—and some women with ADHD flourish in this environment—many women with ADHD find it particularly difficult because it demands self-discipline for focus, time-management, and organization. This challenge is magnified for women who are also parents, as children don't always "get the memo" that mom's trying to work.

Work from Home ADHD Master Plan

To alleviate potential issues and make working from home feasible for you, the following exercise offers research-supported techniques as well as tried-and-true strategies from other women with ADHD.

Instructions

WORK FROM HOME BEST PRACTICES GUIDE

This guide is based off results of a survey conducted on real women with ADHD who work from home in a variety of jobs. Each suggestion is backed by research and tailored to help increase productivity and self-mastery. Many of these strategies can also be tailored for in-office work as well as online schooling or completing coursework at home.

Designate a workspace. When working from home, it can be tempting to open the laptop in any convenient space, like on the bed or a couch. There are many problems with this practice, ranging from a negative impact on productivity to issues with transitioning from work to home life. Instead:

- *Choose a quiet space meant solely for working.* If this is not possible, opt for a temporary workspace, such as an adjustable laptop cart that you can store away after you complete your day.

- *Make it clutter-free and well stocked.* Include everything you'd need in a standard office. Clear your desk before you finish up each day. A clear space can increase your productivity and sense of well-being.

WHAT YOU WILL LEARN

- Strategies and techniques to create a productive work-from-home environment, resulting in improved work satisfaction

WHAT YOU WILL NEED (IN ADDITION TO TIME)

- A designated workspace in your home

ADHD STRENGTHS CREATIVITY, HYPERFOCUS

Change your venue if needed. If you need to be especially productive, find a coffee shop or library where you can focus on your work. There's something about the communal focus of working alongside others that feels contagious and motivating.

Body-double with a co-worker. Work alongside a co-worker (or other friend working from home) through virtual forums. To set up virtual co-working, log into a video chat and place it on mute (to reduce distractions).

Maintain a schedule. Follow the company work schedule, or if you prefer flexibility, set an alternate schedule that you'll follow daily. While a flexible schedule can harness the power of creativity and hyperfocus, it can also lead to burnout and procrastination. To help manage this, women in the survey suggested the following practices for scheduling:

- *Set alarms to signal breaks.* With a lack of external cues from office happenings or co-workers, it can be easy to lose track of time. Set an alarm to take a break every two hours, or however often is needed.

- *Incorporate nourishment.* Hyperfocus can make it difficult to remember routine needs like eating or drinking, and some ADHD medications can further suppress appetite. To address this, set alarms if needed.

- *Block time each week.* At the end of your workweek, identify your most important deadlines for the coming week, and schedule them as appointments in your calendar. You can also time-block publicly as needed. These schedule blocks also keep you accountable to yourself.

CREATE AN ANTI-DISTRACTION SYSTEM

Distractions of any sort can hinder productivity. Setting up barriers to protect your time and space—both physically and virtually—will help prevent issues before they arise. Some actionable ideas include:

Create a do-not-disturb system. This signals to others in your home that you're busy or unavailable. Your system might be as simple as closing the blinds on glass office doors or hanging a sign on the door.

Wear headphones. Try bilateral stimulation music (my favorite is You-Tube's "1 HR Bilateral Music Therapy—Relieve Stress, Anxiety, PTSD, Nervousness—EMDR, Brainspotting" by Destined Dynamics) or color noise therapy, such as brown noise for calming the mind or white noise for improving focus.

Set communication expectations. Tell others how you prefer to be reached and when. Block out times you aren't available and designate times not to respond to emails. This practice prevents a sense of urgency when none is necessary. Turn off notifications on your phone and computer as needed.

Create refocus cues. Write your priority on a sticky note. Place it somewhere visible. If you find yourself distracted, look at the note to remind you what you are working on.

THE POSITIVES

The women surveyed also provided many positives about working from home. By implementing the above best practices, you'll maximize these benefits:

- Flexibility for family time and childcare
- No long commutes
- More agency over meal planning
- Less exposure to office conflict or unnecessary interruptions
- More opportunity for "flow" to occur
- Pajamas . . . enough said!

MOTIVATION

Motivation and follow-through can be among the biggest hurdles for working women with ADHD. Self-blame and frustration around perseverance lead to unrealized potential and keep a woman's gifts and talents locked away. But it doesn't have to be that way. Instead of self-blame, use self-compassion to remember what motivates you.

For increasing motivation, research repeatedly points to the benefits of stimulation and movement. Physical activity instantly improves the ability to focus and the motivation to complete tasks. Based on the research, as little as five minutes of exercise can improve reaction time in our work—meaning every effort counts. Another way to remain motivated is to ensure that you're getting enough mental stimulation. Do this by engaging in challenging tasks and planning your time effectively.

Stay Stimulated

Dopamine works to keep us focused and calm. One of the most efficient ways to naturally increase dopamine and ease restlessness is movement. As a society, we are not encouraged to move enough in our work. Introducing more movement to your work-day can increase productivity, motivation, positive feelings around the work you're doing, and confidence about the work you've completed.

Instructions

PHYSICAL STIMULATION

Physical movement can involve anything—get creative with your movement. Here are a few suggestions:

Try a standing desk. Studies show that standing desks are effective at reducing sedentary behaviors while working and can improve productivity and overall physical health.

Make a date with movement. Choose a time, perhaps at the top of each hour, for least two to five minutes of movement. Whatever you like—walking, dancing, stretching, pushups, jumping jacks—the options are limitless. Look up free workout apps or videos. Fitnessblender.com provides free full-length workouts you can do virtually anywhere.

Fiddle with fidgets. Fidget toys aren't just for kids! You can use this coping tool to your advantage, even in a meeting, by holding a discreet fidget gadget in

WHAT YOU WILL LEARN

- How to get enough mental and physical stimulation through movement and mental challenges to ensure healthy dopamine production
- How stimulation impacts motivation at work

WHAT YOU WILL NEED (IN ADDITION TO TIME)

- A timer or stopwatch
- Space for movement if desired

ADHD STRENGTH ENERGY

your hands (there are countless options to purchase online; however, even a rubber band can work). You might also look into chairs that allow for movement while seated, such as an Upaloop Fitness Seat.

MENTAL STIMULATION

We touched on the Pomodoro Technique in chapter 4. This technique can help keep you motivated. It also ensures you don't hyperfocus for too long, which can cause burnout and issues with motivation. Put it to work for you with these steps:

1. Before starting, consider how long you can work without getting off task. Most women surveyed stated 20 to 30 minutes of working and 5- to 10-minute breaks worked best for them.

2. Plan out what you want to accomplish.

3. Use a timer, or one of the many Pomodoro apps available for your phone, to break your work into intervals separated by short breaks.

4. Save any outside distractions such as emails or other messages for your breaks.

BEATING ADHD PARALYSIS

Shutdown can occur from a long period of overstimulation or hyper-focus. It can also happen when someone with ADHD does not get adequate downtime or alone time, because the ADHD brain needs time to process everything it experiences.

Signs you are reaching this state include:

- Dissociation or brain fog

- Finding it hard to speak or articulate

- Difficulty moving/extreme lethargy

- Inability to tear yourself away from screens, games, puzzles, or books

- Time blindness (page 62)

- Rapid mood and emotional changes

- Difficulty making decisions

- Inability to actively listen

- Jumping from one task to another

- Losing your train of thought

- Anxiety about not getting things done

If you feel this way, try the following strategies:

- Do a daily brain dump. Put tasks in your calendar and eliminate things you don't need to do.

- Focus on completion, not perfection. Setting a time limit on how long you will work on something.

- Schedule rest. It is not wasting time nor is it lazy to relax and recharge.

Chapter Conclusion

Now that you're equipped with new strategies for working, learning, and meeting goals in your life, it is important to remember that you should never feel limited in what you can achieve. When it comes to careers and finding what you want to do, continue to rely on your ability to think creatively. Whether this looks like changing your role in your current job or creating an entirely new business or venture, when you choose to be unique, the possibilities are endless.

Women with ADHD are meant to be seen and heard in the workplace—your gifts have so much to offer. If ever you feel a sense of doubt or find that your symptoms are making your work goals hard to fulfill, know there are ways you can cope. Seeking out opportunities to ground yourself and letting your imagination be free and fluid to come up with your next great idea can help you reengage with your ADHD strengths and abilities. A common space where these grounding moments can be achieved is in our homes, which is why, in the next chapter, we will explore how to make your home as ADHD-friendly as possible, so you can be powered by ADHD in all areas of your life.

Chapter Eight

Home

Home is meant to be your place to feel a sense of safety, well-being, and belonging. For women with ADHD, home life can also elicit shame around keeping up with responsibilities. To create the home you deserve, this chapter explores how to organize efficiently, remain productive, and get ahead of your schedule, so that you can equate home life with relaxation and recovery instead of struggling to keep up.

KEEPING TRACK OF THINGS

Ever notice that when you really need to get out the door on time, you can't find your keys, or wallet, or important papers? Even though you swear you remember where you put them down? This is a common executive function struggle for women with ADHD, especially because they are commonly managing things not only for themselves but for their family as well. In his book *Your Life Can Be Better: Using Strategies for Adult ADD/ADHD*, psychiatrist Douglas Puryear explores how he and his wife used to bicker over him looking past certain items in the refrigerator, even when they were right in front of him.

So why does this happen? There's a social media and pop psychology misconception that those with ADHD suffer from something called **object permanence**, which describes when an individual believes an item or person out of view no longer exists. This is simply not true and is a gross misperception about ADHD. The more accurate reason for things being "out of sight, out of mind" for people with ADHD is due to object retrieval; that is, when the visual cue is not directly in front of them, they have difficulty visualizing and remembering that item, person, or event because of misfiring in working memory centers in the brain. It is a *recall* issue as opposed to a *reality* issue.

To work through object retrieval issues and cut down on time wasted trying to find things, try the simple hack that follows.

A Place for Everything

By creating specific spaces for things in your home, you'll reduce the stress and frustration of trying to recall where things are. The following strategy will save you time and energy while improving efficiency in your home, laying the groundwork for the more involved home hacks offered later in this chapter.

Instructions

1. List any regularly used items needed for your day to run smoothly (examples: medication, keys, phone, wallet, computer, work badge, student ID).

   _____

   _____

   _____

   _____

2. Next, identify the most ideal place for each of these items in your home. If you do not have a designated space, some people like to use a "Doom Box" which stands for: **d**idn't **o**rganize, **o**nly **m**oved and acts as a special container (which for some becomes a drawer or even an entire closet!) that helps people keep track of important items. Though it may be tempting to start using the Doom Box like a "junk" drawer, try to keep it only to important items you need most. You can

WHAT YOU WILL LEARN

- How to eliminate ambiguity and encourage focus around where you put things in your home
- How to reduce time spent on trying to find misplaced things and feel more organized

WHAT YOU WILL NEED (IN ADDITION TO TIME)

- The survey below to set up your initial system
- A writing utensil
- A box if desired

ADHD STRENGTH CREATIVITY

get creative with this by creating a Doom Box that is also visually appealing.

_____

_____

_____

_____

3. Next, move all items to their chosen locations (or Doom Box). Share this location with trusted roommates, partners, or family members, and agree to only place these items in these locations. Set a goal to follow this system for one week to start and then check back on how you did.

4. Allow yourself to release ADHD trauma around shame, and understand that perfection is not the goal, as forming beneficial habits takes time and self-compassion. If you see something out of place, thank yourself for noticing and being mindful and then relocate it as soon as possible. To remind yourself to attend to something right when you first notice it, use the acronym **OHIO: O**nly **H**andle **I**t **O**nce. This is especially useful for the ADHD brain, because the first time we do something, the more interest and energy there is behind it. The more a task is avoided the less motivation there is to complete it.

5. While moving items to specific places in your home, you may get overwhelmed or distracted. One hack includes piling items close to where they go, or en route, and then putting them away when you feel more energized or are on your way there. You might keep "upstairs items" on the side of the steps in a pile. Whenever you head upstairs, grab whatever's there and then (at least) bring it into the room it belongs in. From there, put things in their place before going

to bed each night. One step at a time makes organizing much more manageable.

If you need to hack your hack because you are still struggling, try adding these quick tips:

- Use transparent storage so you can see where things are.

- Make sure your items stand out, such as by adding a bright sticky note or placing them in visible spaces.

- Employ apps when possible, such as a "Find My" phone app. Look into Bluetooth trackers you can use, like an AirTag.

- Take photos of where you put things to refer to later. This can also be very helpful for finding your parking space in a large lot.

ADHD CHALLENGE

CLUTTER

The relationship between ADHD and clutter is complex—some people thrive in a state of "organized chaos," while others feel overwhelmed by their surroundings. Whether you've embraced your creativity within the chaos or are yearning to simplify, there are key elements to thriving with ADHD in a home with a lot of "stuff."

As we've explored, the ADHD brain can be easily distracted by external cues, and every extra item in your space is a cue for attention. With clutter there is just *more*. More to sift through, find, and keep organized. Our homes should serve as a balancing space that grounds us so we can recharge and feel our best in the outside world. To help create the type of home you deserve, the next strategy will look at how creating a regular practice around dealing with clutter can become part of your daily life, as opposed to a major task or obstacle.

The 8-Step Declutter Plan

Try not to look at decluttering as a major project, but rather a habit as normal as brushing your teeth. With regularity, this strategy will become a new way of life. We'll walk through eight steps to decluttering. Take your time and remain positive about any changes you make. You can also tap into your strength of energy by choosing times of the day you are most energized to form your habit around. Whichever you choose, you are still making efforts, and that's what truly matters.

Instructions

Understanding your emotions around clutter can help motivate your efforts. Ask yourself the following questions:

- Am I wasting time looking for what I need?

- Is this searching knocking me off task?

- What areas of my home are the most problematic?

- Do I have conflict with others in my home around clutter?

- Do my children struggle to independently find what they need?

- Do I feel uncomfortable inviting guests into my home?

WHAT YOU WILL LEARN

- How clearing space in your home can help improve ADHD symptoms
- How decluttering can allow for more time and energy to be channeled toward one of your many ADHD strengths

WHAT YOU WILL NEED (IN ADDITION TO TIME)

- A writing utensil
- Disposable trash bags or boxes
- A place to donate items

ADHD STRENGTHS
ENERGY, HYPERFOCUS

Your answers will tell you if clutter is impacting your life. Adapted from an approach created by decluttering expert Dana White, the following eight-step plan can help you successfully declutter and maintain your home.

1. **Choose your focus.** Begin by choosing one space you would like to declutter. Consider areas that are highly used or highly visible to start with so you can enjoy immediate benefits from your effort.

2. **Trash it.** Using a trash bag, get rid of only trash in the designated space. This allows for progress without having to ask yourself too many questions about whether to keep something.

3. **Relocate it.** Bring all items in the space where they truly belong. This allows you to see what is potentially cluttering a space as opposed to what actually belongs there.

4. **Let go.** With all the items remaining, ask yourself if there is anything you can donate or let go of. This step can lead to strong emotions for some, and many individuals find this is where they get stuck (if you can relate, see "How to Let Things Go," page 86).

5. **Trust your instincts.** When organizing, try not to think about where others would put something, but rather where you instinctually would look for this item first. The more you honor your natural instincts, the better your space will work for you.

6. **Respect spatial boundaries.** Contain or organize everything, making use of what you have without spreading into new storage. For example, if you have socks spilling out of your drawer, don't buy another container to put the extra socks; instead, keep your favorites and let go of the rest. (Hint: The socks on the top layer are most likely your favorites.)

7. **Put things away.** Try your best to finish that space entirely and bring things where they belong at that very moment. If you can't finish now, block out an appointment on your calendar to finish the job.

8. **Use ADHD-friendly organization.** When you put things away:

- Circle back to O.H.I.O. (on page 80).

- Put unmanageable clutter, such as wires or electronics, in one clear container for storage.

- When choosing spaces for things, consider how the overall space looks.

- Place things together where you'll most likely use them.

- Use clear containers or labels whenever possible.

- Use Marie Kondo's vertical folding technique so items are easier to find. For example, imagine your pants stacked in a row, as you would stack books with spines facing out, but inside a drawer.

KEEP YOUR SPACE CLEAR LONG-TERM

This approach is not a one-time event—it's an ongoing routine. Start with small successes and witness your progress over time. Here's how to keep it going:

- Set a timer for at least five minutes each day to declutter what you can.

- Never leave your car without something in your hand. The idea is to clear your car out every time you drive as opposed to letting clutter build up.

- Keep a bag for donations available at all times. As soon as the container is full, put it in a handy location (like the front seat of your car) and donate it within a week.

- Begin with small projects you can complete fully (like your purse as opposed to a playroom). The positive reinforcement that comes from task completion helps inspire long-term change.

HOW TO LET THINGS GO

If you have a hard time letting go of "stuff," consider these two strategies from the experts:

Strategy 1: "The Minimalists" podcasters, Joshua Fields Millburn and Ryan Nicodemus, suggest asking yourself:

- Can I replace this item for less than twenty dollars?

- Can I replace this item in less than twenty minutes?

   If the answer is "yes," let it go.

Strategy 2: Organization expert Marie Kondo suggests exploring whether something "sparks joy" for you:

1. Feel the item in your hand.

2. Notice how your body reacts when holding it.

3. If it feels as if your entire body is lifted, this indicates the spark of joy.

4. If the item instead makes you feel depleted, lowered, tired, or drained, then this item does not spark joy, and Kondo suggests letting it go.

   Choosing to express gratitude to the item for the purpose it served, donating it, or selling it are all wonderful ways to complete the cycle of owning an item.

SCHEDULING

One of the most frustrating struggles for women with ADHD is managing time, and it can be even more difficult for women with families. Missed appointments, chronic lateness, double-booking, missed opportunities, or forgotten events are just some of the frustrating consequences of not keeping a schedule that works. Self-confidence can suffer as a result, causing feelings of inadequacy and overwhelm.

Mastering Your Schedule

WHAT YOU WILL LEARN

- Potential pitfalls in your current method of scheduling

- How to create an effective system you can stick to

WHAT YOU WILL NEED (IN ADDITION TO TIME)

- Your planner of choice

- A timer and journal for recording

ADHD STRENGTH CREATIVITY

ADHD symptoms can hamper efforts to manage an effective schedule. By learning ways to master your schedule at home, you'll likely find that time management becomes easier in other areas of your life as well. The following strategy implements time awareness, which will help you create an effective schedule and understand how to sustain these efforts long-term.

Instructions

1. **Find out how much time things *actually* take you.** Time blindness makes it difficult to witness the passing of time, as well as to know how much time is needed to complete a task. Podcaster and ADHD coach Eric Tivers shares an important strategy:

   a. Set a stopwatch to start counting up when you begin a task. The time should include setup for the task, doing the task, and cleaning up or ending the task.

   b. See how long the task took, as many of us underestimate how much time we truly need.

2. **Choose your calendar.** This calendar should be easily accessible. Most of my clients use a virtual calendar, but some enjoy using a paper planner, which they take with them everywhere. For home and family, you can share virtual calendars or put

up a massive whiteboard calendar in the kitchen, so literally no one can miss it.

3. **Color code it.** Get creative by making unique visual cues on the calendar for each person, such as a different color for each family member. Within my own, I even have multiple colors, depending on what type of event it is (for example, writing blocks are yellow, counseling is purple, and personal events are green).

4. **Choose what goes on the calendar.** Begin with appointments and firm commitments. Block those (as well as travel time) out first. If something is highly critical or there is prep work leading up to an event, you can set reminders at intervals of your choice. For example, when writing this book, I had numerous deadlines to meet. I marked my calendar for every Tuesday to check in on my progress leading up to these deadlines.

5. **Identify your IBNUs**. IBNU (**i**mportant **b**ut **n**ot **u**rgent) events are things you want to accomplish but don't necessarily have to do (such as exercise, meditation, date nights, or hobbies). Some people with ADHD balk at the idea of a schedule, as they don't like feeling constrained; however, your calendar can be flexible when you need it to be. Many women struggle to set aside time for themselves, but when it is blocked out, they find they have time to focus on their IBNUs. Blocking time in this visual way increases awareness and can provide a sense of accomplishment.

6. **Create a ritual.** Check your calendar daily and review it at the start and end of the day to prepare you for what lies ahead. Integrate this habit with another ritual by **habit stacking**, which is when you pair a habit you already have with one you are trying to establish (such as taking your morning medication when you brush your teeth).

7. **Ask for support.** If you share a home with others, engage them all in the calendar so you're not the sole person aware of what's to come.

If you are single, you can share your calendar with a trusted friend, or invite others to events and include them on a shared virtual calendar so you both see it.

As you work to master your schedule, life may get in the way. Try not to be hard on yourself or reinforce old failure narratives. Instead, remember that everyone, not just those with ADHD, becomes overwhelmed with scheduling their busy lives. Continued efforts to be mindful of your schedule will help lessen frustration around time management. And remember, self-compassion and repetition are key to making these new habits stick.

CHORES

A common struggle for maintaining a home with ADHD is keeping up with the endless responsibilities of household chores. Many women I work with feel as if they are *always* doing them, which is true. For example, chores like laundry are never truly "done." Rather, we are in a perpetual cycle: clothes being worn, clothes being washed, clothes being put away. To think that chores have a finish line can cause a false narrative that feeds a story of failure. Conversely, finding a way to be in rhythm with this cycle can be empowering.

Chore-Tackling Plan

WHAT YOU WILL LEARN

- Why chores are a common issue for those with ADHD
- How to create and maintain a clean and organized home without stress

WHAT YOU WILL NEED (IN ADDITION TO TIME)

- A calendar or planner
- A writing utensil

ADHD STRENGTHS
ENERGY, HYPERFOCUS

With ADHD, having systems in place for chores can be a game-changer. It'll make the mountain of tasks feel more manageable and leave you feeling more energized and accomplished. The following exercise explores the most common reasons someone with ADHD struggles with chores and specific techniques that real women with ADHD use to address these challenges. From there, you'll be prompted to create a personalized Chore-Tackling Plan to make chores feel more manageable.

Instructions

1. **If you feel overwhelmed:**

   Enlist help. Historically, women were responsible for chores in the home and were not encouraged to ask for help. For many, it still seems to be the case. This is simply not sustainable nor is it fair. You have the right to engage partners, children, and roommates in the sharing of household duties, and if they are not supporting you, then there is a much larger conversation to be had. If financially possible, another option is to hire out-side help.

   Try not to overcommit. Instead of leaving every-thing to a single "cleaning day" (which serves a different purpose, such as preparing for a big event or getting more detailed in a cleaning process—and may work well for some), it's less overwhelming to do a little each day.

Use smart storage. Keep cleaning supplies in the spaces they are needed. For example, store rags and cleaning products under the sink, and keep a trash bag in your car. Having things within arm's reach will prevent you from getting distracted by other things when you're doing a chore. This skill can be used to streamline virtually anything in your house.

Embrace self-compassion. Remain focused on what you've accomplished and let go of what hasn't been done so you can take care of your emotional needs. And take breaks. Try setting an alarm for 10 minutes and read, meditate, take a hot shower, or do anything else that grounds you. Or have these moments of rest be the reward once you get the chores completed.

2. **If you tend to forget certain chores:**

Use your calendar or planner. Block off chores for each day, including how long you expect that task to take (perhaps timing yourself as described in the previous skill). You might choose to stick to one category per day, such as tidying two adjacent rooms or focusing on the entire bathroom.

Habit stack. For example, after you clean the dishes from dinner, always check the mail.

Set reminders. Using alarms can help enforce your new routine.

Use a highly visible chore chart. This provides a visual cue of what needs to be done. It can also provide positive reinforcement when you cross off an item. Use the Chore-Tackling Plan in this exercise, purchase one, or create your own. And check it daily.

3. **If you get bored doing chores:**

   Listen to music. Use headphones or play it throughout your home.

   Listen to an audiobook or podcast. Keeping mentally engaged can occupy you and even encourage a state of hyperfocus so you're not as fixated on the drudgery of the chore.

   Talk to a friend. Do this on speaker or use Bluetooth headphones to keep your hands free.

   Make it competitive. Challenge a family member or housemate to see who can finish their task first. With your gift of energy, you have an excellent advantage!

The following Chore-Tackling Plan highlights common chores and includes empty spaces for you to add any other chores. From the techniques you just read, choose the ones you think would work best, as well as when you plan to do each chore. To ensure success, block out these chores in your calendar.

When you miss a chore (because no one is perfect), try not to get into a self-blame cycle! Instead, revisit your Chore-Tackling Plan to get back on track. You may find that some ideas work better than others, so continue to try new approaches until some of them stick.

CHORE	WHEN AND HOW OFTEN?	WHO IS RESPONSIBLE?	SKILL(S) FOR FEELING OVERWHELMED	SKILL(S) FOR MY ROUTINE	SKILL(S) TO COMBAT BOREDOM
Bedroom(s)					
Bathroom(s)					
Floors					
Decluttering					
Car					
Dishes					
Kid prep					
Laundry					
Kitchen					
Mail					

Chapter Conclusion

A home that feels clear and balanced can also be a holistic form of treatment for ADHD. The less stuff you have, the less work and cleaning there is, and the less decision-making you need to do daily. As you continue to engage in these helpful techniques, there will be more opportunities for your ADHD gifts to unfold. The best way to keep a sense of balance in your home is by making a daily commitment to practice the skills learned in this chapter. Also remember the importance of teamwork and enlisting help from others in your home, as the entirety of managing your home should not fall solely on your shoulders.

Chapter 9
Finances

For people with ADHD, budgeting and finances can be an overwhelming topic to explore. You may feel like you're just "not good with money." Effective budgeting involves self-control and future planning, which aren't always easy, and for the more creative and spontaneous ADHD brain, issues around finances can increase anxiety. The good news is that there are effective ways for those with ADHD to improve their finances, which will allow for more freedom to explore life and tap into the many gifts ADHD has to offer.

BUDGETING

Many women with ADHD struggle with finances because traditional forms of budgeting do not always work for them. Shame around not remembering to pay bills or having a skewed perception around the ability to pay off debt, creates what experts call the "ADHD tax." This refers to the extra effort, resources, and time people with ADHD must put into tasks that are often much easier for others. This extra effort makes it more difficult to become financially secure and can cost those with ADHD more money in the form of late charges and higher interest rates. Despite the grim picture painted, awareness is the first step in learning how to overcome financial struggles. Women with ADHD, just like anyone else, can budget effectively, and the following exercise will show you how.

Powered by ADHD Budgeting Plan

This exercise will teach you what to focus on when creating and maintaining an ADHD-friendly budget. These were also explored on Jessica McCabe's *How to ADHD* YouTube channel episode, "How to Fix Your Credit (and How ADHD Gets in the Way)." These steps are meant to override potential pitfalls when it comes to finances, such as forgetfulness or impulsivity, while remaining in charge of your financial choices. While this strategy will take time to produce positive growth, lasting changes are possible when you commit to the ideas that follow.

Instructions

1. **Automate everything.** With ADHD, the more you can automate in life the better. One of the reasons budgeting, balancing a checkbook, or using an elaborate financial app does not always work for those with ADHD is that it requires action on your part. Automation helps improve executive functioning around organization, planning, and short-term memory issues that can prevent you from paying your bills on time. Here's how to put this step into practice:

   - Set up auto-pay on all possible bills.

   - If you need to direct money to certain accounts for bills, set up auto-draft ahead of time.

WHAT YOU WILL LEARN

- A three-step plan for ADHD-friendly budgeting
- Plan variations that account for impulsivity and distractibility

WHAT YOU WILL NEED (IN ADDITION TO TIME)

- Access to accounts and bills
- Your calendar or alarm system used for reminders

ADHD STRENGTH CREATIVITY

- If there are bills you cannot automate, set alarms, notifications, or reminders at least one day ahead to pay the bill. You can get creative with reminders by using certain audio cues for certain bills or even creating visual reminders in your calendar.

- Set up automated low-balance alerts on your banking app to alert you if your balance falls below a certain amount.

2. **Build a safety net.** Studies show that those with ADHD are less likely to have enough in savings and more likely to spend the money they do have. A safety net can be vital in a time of crisis (such as losing a job or your car breaking down). A safety net also comes in handy when an opportunity arises, such as a friend's destination wedding or the chance to engage in a new hobby. While saving money may seem restricting and quite possibly the opposite of enjoyable, it allows for freedom when unexpected moments arise. Here's how to put this step into practice:

- Use the snowball method: once you pay off a smaller bill, put the money that once went toward that bill into savings.

- Search your bank statements for subscriptions or services you are no longer using. Once you cancel them, take the money you were spending on them and funnel it into your savings.

- If you get a raise or a new job with higher pay, transfer the difference into your savings. Some call this "paying yourself first," meaning the money is no longer available in your account to pay others (or to buy things) but rather it is paid into your safety net.

3. **Prevent impulse spending.** While automation works wonderfully for saving or paying bills, it has the opposite effect for spending. Have you seen those videos about going to Target for "one thing" and leaving 200 dollars and two hours later bleary-eyed and unsure what just happened? To overcome impulse spending, put systems

into place that make it less convenient for you to spend money. As you do this, also encourage self-compassion and mindfulness around making purchases. Recent research found that self-compassion increased self-control in instances of spending, as well as reducing materialism. Utilize these practical steps:

- Create a shopping list and stick to it.

- Shop for groceries online and pick them up curbside, or have them delivered (the delivery fee will more than offset the cost of any impulse items you might have otherwise bought).

- Choose your budget before shopping. For example, if you are looking for a gift, decide on the price point first and try to stay within the limit.

- Remove any credit card information stored on online shopping sites, and use your debit card so you know you're only spending money you have.

- Delete frequently used shopping apps from your phone. The ease at which we are able to spend is highly problematic when trying to curb impulse spending, and any extra steps between shopping and purchasing result in more intentional consideration.

- Pause between the urge and action—the longer you wait, the better. If any part of you feels uncertain about a purchase, remove it from your cart and come back to it later. By then, you may have lost the impulse to buy it, changed your mind, or forgotten about it altogether.

CREDIT

Your credit and credit score tell a story about how you have managed your finances over time, informing lenders whether you qualify for loans, and if you do, whether you receive fair rates. A good credit score is not dependent on your income or wealth, but rather how you manage what you have. Research shows that those with ADHD begin adulthood with adequate credit scores and default rates (the percentage of outstanding loans written off as unpaid or having prolonged periods of missed payments); yet by middle age, their default rates grow, causing their credit scores to suffer in comparison to non-ADHD adults of the same age. You have the power to change your credit score over time—this strategy will show you how.

Credit-Boosting Skills

This strategy provides eight helpful steps to improve your credit score. It might help to schedule blocks of time to work on any disputes, issues, or payment of bills. Improving your credit score does take time, but every effort you make will have a positive impact in the long term.

Instructions

Before you start, find out your credit score. Choose a website or app, such as creditkarma.com or experian.com, which are especially useful for setting up automated alerts on your score. From there, you can start to work toward your desired score (or maintain or increase the one you have already) by doing the following:

1. **Don't miss payments.** Using your calendar, identify when payments are due and make sure all of them are up to date. Set as many up for auto-pay as possible.

2. **Keep balances low.** Keeping credit card balances below 30 percent of the credit available is important; anything above this can negatively impact your score. You may want to pay more on the higher cards first. This contradicts some financial advice saying pay off the smaller bills first, but the priority here is improving credit).

3. **Check for errors.** Duplicate charges or balance errors can hurt your credit score. If you find any,

WHAT YOU WILL LEARN

- Which methods are most effective for improving your credit score
- Practical ways to put these methods to use immediately

WHAT YOU WILL NEED (IN ADDITION TO TIME)

- A preferred app or website to check your credit score
- Contact information for the credit bureau if needed
- Login information for your credit card companies and accounts

contact the credit bureau as soon as possible at any of the following numbers:

- Experian (888) 397-3742

- TransUnion (800) 916-8800

- Equifax (866) 349-5191

It can take 30 to 45 days for them to investigate and respond, so consider setting up a follow-up call on your calendar to check in.

4. **Use credit responsibly.** Your score is based on effective handling of finances, so use your card for non-impulse purchases such as gas and pay it off monthly. However, not using the card at all doesn't help your score.

5. **Avoid opening multiple accounts in a short time.** Lenders look at the age and history of your accounts, and younger accounts yield a lower score value. Also, you must maintain open cards to build credit on them, so you don't want to take on more accounts than you can handle.

6. **Try not to close credit card accounts.** This can impact your credit score. However, do not overspend or use your cards when you cannot afford it. The best option is to strategically use your cards for required expenses and pay them off as soon as possible.

7. **Try searching for loans during short time periods.** When applying for loans or a new account, you continue to get "soft hits" on your credit, which is not detrimental to your score unless there is high activity over a length of time.

8. **Get added as an authorized user on another person's card.** This can help you establish credit history and build your credit—just be careful that they themselves make responsible financial choices, since their actions on this card will affect you.

IMPULSE SPENDING

There are many reasons why we spend. According to NerdWallet, the most common emotions connected to impulse spending are stress, anxiety, and sadness. And the world sure makes it easy to spend. From engaging and delicious impulse items conveniently located by the checkout register, to targeted ads for products "we can't live without" leaping through our screens into our personal space (that were curated specifically based on our online browsing habits), savvy marketing experts know just how to reach us and our emotions.

Unfortunately, impulse shopping can become habitual and damage our credit and even our sense of peace and control. But when we start to pay attention to why we spend money, we can learn to curb impulsive spending before it begins. Feeling in control in this area can also help alleviate negative self-talk. Since everyone's financial situation is unique, the following exercise will help you gain insight into your personal spending style.

Gain Control Over Impulse Purchases

When trying to reduce the use of an unhealthy coping skill, such as impulse spending, it's helpful to gain insight into why we do it. As mentioned, negative emotions can motivate impulse purchases, but positive emotions, celebrations, and events can do the same. The following questionnaire will provide insight into what motivates your spending habits, then we'll introduce some ADHD-friendly skills that can help you gain control over what and when you spend.

WHAT YOU WILL LEARN

- What's motivating your impulse purchases
- When you are most likely to spend
- How to lessen impulse spending

WHAT YOU WILL NEED (IN ADDITION TO TIME)

- This book or a journal
- A writing utensil

Instructions

Ask yourself the following questions and write down your response to each one:

1. Are there certain events, holidays, or times of year when I spend the most?

   _____

   _____

   _____

2. During these times or events, what (or whom) am I spending the most on?

   _____

   _____

   _____

   _____

3. Do I ever make purchases late at night or when I'm tired?

_____

_____

_____

4. Do I ever regret purchases? If so, what, typically, are these purchases?

_____

_____

_____

5. Do I have a difficult time saying no to others when they ask me to do or buy things that cost more than my means? If yes, who do I find it the hardest to say no to?

_____

_____

_____

_____

6. Do I spend a great deal on DIY projects that I think will save me money, but in the end do not?

_____

_____

_____

_____

7. How do I feel when I make an impulse purchase?

_____

_____

_____

_____

Take a moment to read through your answers and consider the main themes around when and why you spend. Checking in with yourself is an important step in stopping any unhealthy patterns. The dopamine released from spending can make us feel wonderful, for a very short amount of time, or until we spend again. Because of the addictive nature of spending money, some people find having a support person, coach, or financial planner helps keep them accountable. No matter how you approach this, remember the key budgeting tips to stop impulse spending:

- Use shopping lists and stick to them.

- If you can, order your groceries online.

- Create budgets for gifts or focused shopping.

- Remove your credit card information from online merchants.

- Delete frequently used shopping apps.

- Give yourself time to mindfully decide before you buy.

- Check in with your emotions around a purchase before checking out.

Chapter Conclusion

Having ADHD doesn't mean you will necessarily struggle with finances. Many women have found financial success and freedom, and you can too. By figuring out which budgeting methods work for you, keeping up with your credit score, and paying attention to impulse spending, you can greatly improve this area of your life. In doing so, you have the potential to become further powered by your ADHD, as with financial freedom you have the means to become more engaged in all the things your ADHD brain wishes to explore.

Chapter Ten

Parenting

Parenting is a dynamic journey, packed with some of the most fulfilling moments, as well as some of the most challenging ones. When parenting with ADHD, especially if left untreated, feeling overwhelmed can become a more frequent occurrence. This chapter explores how to make parenting with ADHD more manageable and rewarding, by balancing self-care with caring for others.

Even if you are not yet a parent, or do not plan on becoming one, this chapter offers ideas around healthy boundaries in a variety of caretaking relationships. Women who are in a helping profession or care for elderly parents will find some of the skills relatable, and new mothers will get some guidance in navigating ADHD during pregnancy, birth, and the postpartum phase.

PREGNANCY

Pregnancy can be one of the most exciting times in a woman's life—as well as being ridden with anxiety and uncertainty. There's so much to plan and think about: how your life will change after the baby arrives, what kind of birth you want to have, whether you will continue working outside the home, or, for those who will become a single parent, what that might look like. Pregnancy can impact women with ADHD in unique ways. We'll consider challenges such as mental or physical health issues, work and vocational demands, and family dynamics whether it is your first pregnancy or a subsequent one. In the end, you are the expert of your experience, and only you can determine what you need. So, take what you will from this chapter and choose what works for you, and let it help enrich your parenting journey.

ADHD Pregnancy Guide

The following guide explores common issues that arise while managing ADHD throughout various stages of pregnancy. Hormonal changes and pregnancy's impact on executive functioning are common risk factors for pregnant women with ADHD as well as is the increased risk of struggling with mental health disorders. This guide also contains tips and strategies for optimizing your physical and mental health during pregnancy.

WHAT YOU WILL LEARN

- What challenges pregnant women with ADHD commonly face
- How to navigate challenges and get the support you need from those around you.

ADHD STRENGTHS
ENERGY, SPONTANEITY

Early stages of pregnancy. At conception, significant hormonal shifts support the health of the developing baby. Hormones such as estrogen, human chorionic gonadotropin (HCG), and progesterone all increase as they support the baby's growth, while simultaneously wreaking havoc on the pregnant woman's physical and mental well-being. All of this can make navigating pregnancy with ADHD quite challenging. Changes in estrogen are also linked to anxiety, depression, and irritability, while progesterone can increase feelings of anxiety or sadness. Early detection of any depression symptoms is critical, so you can get the support you need to function at your best.

   Symptoms of depression during pregnancy include:

- Frequent sadness or crying

- Diminished interest in becoming a mother

- Feeling worthless or guilty, especially about not being a good mother

- Strong anxiety, tension, and/or fear

- Sleep problems not associated with the physical discomfort of pregnancy (not being able to sleep or sleeping more than usual but not feeling rested)

- Diminished energy

- Trouble focusing, remembering things, or making decisions

- Feeling restless or irritable

- Headaches, chest pains, heart palpitations, numbness, or hyperventilation

- Suicidal thoughts

To further complicate the issue, a rise in estrogen can also cause feelings of bliss and well-being, causing an upswing in mood and accounting for what we call the "highs and lows" of pregnancy. Even though these mood swings are normal, they can be difficult to navigate. For this reason, support is crucial for both mother and baby.

Every emotion you experience is valid and deserves a safe space to be expressed. It is important to share how you are feeling with a supportive partner, medical provider, friends, or family. Anyone who you feel invalidates or minimizes your experience probably does not understand the nature of what it means to be pregnant with ADHD. If this happens, invite them to read this section of the book, or you may want to seek out a more supportive outlet for your concerns.

Self-care is perhaps the greatest gift you can give yourself and your unborn baby, to manage your mood while pregnant and is most likely to help encourage your continued ADHD strength of energy through pregnancy. Here are some beneficial self-care strategies:

Move as much as possible. Most physical activity you did before pregnancy is usually safe to continue during pregnancy, but always check first with your medical provider. Some common ways to move that women enjoy doing during pregnancy include:

- Prenatal yoga and Pilates
- Swimming
- Walking and hiking
- Riding a stationary bike or elliptical
- Resistance training
- Low-impact aerobics

Find community. Whether this is your first or fifth pregnancy, it's vital to have a sense of support. Motivation to find a new community can be supported by your gift of spontaneity and wanting to try new things and meet new people. To do so you can join an online (or in-person) support group to process your experiences and emotions with other women who are pregnant and even those with ADHD. I loved the *What to Expect* online forums. Also remember that people who care about you also want to be part of your community of support, even if they aren't pregnant or don't have ADHD.

Eat well. Eating serotonin-boosting foods you can tolerate while pregnant will help regulate your mood, improve your sleep, and help lift brain fog. Eat small, regularly spaced meals often throughout the day to stabilize your blood sugar and ward off nausea caused by hormonal fluctuations. Some mood-boosting foods include:

- Eggs
- Bananas
- Nuts
- Dark chocolate
- Dairy products
- Unprocessed tofu
- Low-mercury fish
- Whole grains
- Green tea

ADHD MEDICATION DURING PREGNANCY

According to the Centers for Disease Control and Prevention, an increasing number of pregnant women are taking ADHD medication.

In a study conducted by the National Birth Defects Prevention Study, researchers explored the prevalence of women taking ADHD medication during pregnancy, as well as links between ADHD medication and birth defects in babies. The study found the number of women who continued ADHD medication during pregnancy doubled from 1998 to 2011. Of those who continue medication use, there was an increased risk of birth defects; however, the risk was determined to be minimal.

Discuss your options with a medical provider who has in-depth knowledge of perinatal psychiatry and adult ADHD, and who will consider your unique symptoms and circumstances. Some women opt to discontinue medication until pregnancy is over, or longer if planning to breastfeed. Others choose to reduce ADHD medication dosage to the lowest tolerated dose. Some doctors recommend changing your current prescription from a Class D to Class C ADHD medication, if another medication is a viable option.

Class C medications: Adderall, Zenzedi, and Focalin. Animal reproduction studies have shown an adverse effect on the fetus; however, there are no adequate and well-controlled studies on humans.

Class D medications: Methylphenidate and Ritalin. There is positive evidence of human fetal risk based on adverse reaction data from investigational or marketing experience or studies on humans.

In both cases, potential benefits may outweigh potential risks, depending on the individual.

No matter what medication route you choose, the decision is yours alone. While it's important to consider your partner in the decision process, your body and mental health are most impacted, now and after birth.

POSTPARTUM ADJUSTMENT

After birth, some women report their ADHD symptoms worsen, especially during the first six weeks postpartum. There's a lot going on: hormones plummeting, any physical trauma (especially from a C-section) or birth complications, lack of sleep, as well as changes that occur in a new mother's brain and limbic system. Studies show that areas of the limbic system, especially the amygdala, change to help the new mother (and even other primary caregivers who are highly involved!) become hypervigilant to their surroundings. This hypervigilance leads to distractibility that can impact other executive functions, further intensifying ADHD symptoms.

ADHD Postpartum Guide

There's an age-old saying that babies should come with a manual. Luckily, many mothers have walked this path before you, including countless moms with ADHD, and there is an entire world of support and knowledge out there for you to tap into. Hopefully, you have been and will continue reading, learning, and reaching out to your support system. To build on this knowledge, this strategy will provide some ADHD-specific insights to help you effectively navigate the first six months.

WHAT YOU WILL LEARN

- Common postpartum issues and how to respond

- Wellness goals you can work toward for optimal feelings of physical and mental well-being

ADHD STRENGTH
ENERGY

POSTPARTUM WELLNESS

The postpartum period can be divided into three distinct stages:

- Initial or acute phase, 8 to 19 hours after childbirth

- Subacute postpartum period, which lasts 2 to 6 weeks

- Delayed postpartum period, which can last up to 6 months

Each phase poses its own challenges. Use this time as best you can to recover so you can manage your ADHD symptoms and overall wellness. Granted, that can be easier said than done when you're caring for a needy newborn! But your gift of energy can help support this journey and enhance your well-being, which is as important as that of your baby.

POSTPARTUM DEPRESSION

According to the National Institutes of Health, around one in every seven women can suffer from postpartum depression. Symptoms may include:

- Depressed mood or severe mood swings

- Intense irritability

- Sadness or excessive crying

- Difficulty concentrating

- Difficulty bonding with your baby

- Fear that you're not a good mother

- Sleep issues (too much or too little)

- Exhaustion or reduced energy

- Shame or feelings of not being enough

- Severe anxiety or panic attacks

- Eating issues (too much or too little)

- Withdrawal from loved ones

- Recurring thoughts of death or suicide

If you believe you may be experiencing PPD, or if you feel like you might harm yourself or your baby, reach out to your doctor and enlist your support system right away. This is one reason that surrounding yourself with supportive people is so important—so you can have a safe person to check in with if needed. PPD is common and treatable. Nobody should have to suffer through PPD without help. You may be too focused on your baby to worry about yourself, but you will be able to care better for your baby when your basic needs are met too.

10 DAILY POSTPARTUM WELLNESS GOALS

1. Take your vitamins

2. Hydrate (64 ounces—herbal tea and watery fruits and veggies count!)

3. Move your body

4. Shower and dress—which helps provide healthy stimulation and structure to your day

5. Go outdoors

6. Rest with meditation or a nap

7. Read something inspiring

8. Nourish yourself with good food

9. Journal your experience (this can also help with noticing any unhealthy feelings or patterns)

10. Spend time with a supportive person (even if just on the phone)

Many of these daily goals can be done with your baby and serve as quality time, while also modeling healthy coping skills for other children in the home. Some mothers also report issues with excessive worry after childbirth (and adoption), and they describe themselves as feeling constantly nervous or panicked. In this case, postpartum anxiety may be the issue and similar wellness goals can help alleviate these symptoms as well.

PARENTAL BURNOUT

Parental burnout presents as a chronic state of exhaustion that can develop in people with ADHD when executive functioning skills and focus occur over a long period of time without any breaks. Burnout often occurs when there are excessive levels of stress while parenting and stress becomes chronic, which is more common with ADHD.

Common signs of parental burnout:

- Increased yelling, outbursts, or conflicts with children or others
- Detachment or withdrawal from people or activities
- Recurrent guilty feelings about parenting or negative interactions
- Lingering grudges or resentments toward children
- Negative thinking
- Frustration and irritability
- Anxiety and stress symptoms
- Depression symptoms, including hopelessness
- Sleep difficulties
- Unhealthy coping behaviors
- Feelings of inadequacy or self-hatred
- Changes in appetite or sleep habits
- Persistent feelings of exhaustion
- Physical health problems caused by stress
- Avoidance of parenting duties
- Headaches or gastrointestinal distress

For those with ADHD, additional signs:

- Feeling overwhelmed or wanting to escape
- Declining productivity and performance
- Reduced self-confidence
- Lower self-esteem, feeling incompetent, lazy, or incapable
- Lack of motivation or energy
- Feeling angry or resentful
- Increased irritability, mood swings, or emotional extremes
- Procrastinating or avoiding people, obligations, or tasks
- Taking more time than normal to complete basic tasks
- Increased substance use

Overcoming Parental Burnout

WHAT YOU WILL LEARN

- How to lead with self-compassion rather than self-blame so you can care for yourself and others

WHAT YOU WILL NEED (IN ADDITION TO TIME)

- A writing utensil
- This book or a journal

ADHD STRENGTHS
SPONTANEITY, ENERGY, CREATIVITY

This strategy will provide you with specific ways to engage in self-care and get your needs met while still effectively parenting. The section will conclude with an opportunity to create your own Anti-Burnout Plan.

Instructions

Start with gratitude. Being grateful for what is causing you stress is not always the most intuitive thing to do when overcoming burnout. However, purposeful gratitude causes a positive shift in your perspective. Researchers and psychologists have found that practicing gratitude over time can actually change your personality and mood for the better. Here are specific ways to use gratitude to reduce parental burnout:

List your child's strengths. Refocus on what you appreciate about your children. It can also help manage expectations and compassion for your children if they also have ADHD.

Smile. Smiling sends positive signals to the brain and can lessen the feeling of burnout. Even a *half smile* can relax your body and mind. To do so, relax your face from your forehead down to your jaw and chin, and turn the corns of your lips upwards ever so slightly. Your brain will read this as an invitation to relax.

Notice the positive. Positive psychologists, who study human strengths and virtues, state that happiness is not based on achieving what we want, but rather on being grateful for what we have. Whether you write it down in a journal, tap into your creativity by creating art around gratitude (such as the grateful pumpkin my family did this fall), or practice saying one thing you're grateful for at the dinner table, the simple practice of noticing the positive can help reduce burnout and negative feelings.

Make repair attempts. A repair attempt is any statement or action—verbal, physical, or otherwise (such as tickling, telling a joke, or doing something relaxing together)—that is meant to defuse negativity and conflict. So, turn some music on, grab your child's hand and start dancing.

Practice self-compassion. Allow yourself freedom to feel however you need to. Speak to yourself as you would a friend. Radically accepting the hard parts, while reducing the desire to criticize with shame, can help lessen the mental load you're already carrying. Have patience when practicing self-compassion, and maintain a "growth mindset"; that is, believe that conflicts provide an opportunity to learn and grow as a parent and family.

Because burnout affects everyone differently, recovery time can vary from weeks to even months or years. In essence, it's about balancing *energy out* with *energy in*. To take what you have learned about managing ADHD parental burnout, use the following exercise to set goals to prevent burnout in the present or future.

ANTI-BURNOUT PLAN

Check off each activity that appeals to you, and add any other things that bring you joy or peace (this is an area where your gifts of energy and spontaneity can help support your progress). Then, complete the plan for how you will use these skills.

— Exercise

— Meditate/pray

— Create something

— Journal

— Do something fun with your children

— Do something fun for yourself

— Take a bubble bath

— Ask your partner for help

— Ask others for help

— Go on a date with your partner

— Go on a date with yourself

— Spend time with or call a friend

— Practice gratitude

— Nap

— Watch a movie

— Go outdoors

— Practice yoga, tai chi, or other energy-moving practices

— Practice breath work

— Practice self-compassion

— See live music

— Dance

— Other:

_____

_____

_____

I will do the following daily:

_____

_____

_____

_____

I will do the following weekly:

_____

_____

_____

I will do the following monthly:

_____

_____

_____

I will ask for support to make this plan possible by speaking to:

_____

_____

_____

The best days and times for me to engage in these coping skills:

_____

_____

_____

Make follow-through more likely by scheduling each of these on your calendar!

MOTIVATION HACK

Sometimes it seems impossible to motivate action, especially when you are stressed. In this case, you can push through the motivation wall by hijacking your brain with a popular social media hack.

1. If part of you wants to get moving but the other part wants to procrastinate and do nothing, give yourself a short period of time to relax (perhaps 30 minutes or less).

2. Using a timer or alarm, set the time for the end of the procrastination period and move the alarm far enough away from you that you'll have to get up when it goes off. Better yet, place the alarm near your goal—for example, set it on top of your home treadmill if the goal is to work out.

3. When the alarm goes off, you'll have to get up and move toward your goal (unless you can stand listening to an endless alarm!).

4. Choose to end the procrastination period now that you are up. If you like, reset the alarm for when you will stop performing your task.

GENERATIONAL ADHD

Nearly half of children with ADHD have parents with the diagnosis. When generational ADHD occurs, it's important for parents to begin with self-compassion and manage their own ADHD, so they can model healthy ways of navigating executive functioning challenges while still setting realistic expectations for their children. Learning ways to use your ADHD traits as strengths in parenting will empower you and your children and make parenting with ADHD easier and more rewarding.

ADHD Parenting Hacks

Much like parenting a child with ADHD, parents with ADHD need to provide themselves with adequate structure and routine to balance their own responsibilities without becoming overwhelmed or burnt out. The following strategy offers 9 practical, solution-focused parenting hacks to help make parenting with ADHD feel more manageable.

Note: There are a number of ideas presented in this section. To avoid feeling overwhelmed, select a few to get started with. Once they become habits, choose another.

Instructions

1. **Mealtime.** Studies show that families who eat meals together show greater synchronicity and improved communication. Other benefits include resilience, higher self-esteem, greater academic performance, and lower instances of youth mental health and eating disorders and substance abuse. To make mealtime more manageable:

   - Cook meals ahead with an Instant Pot or Crock-Pot.

   - Meal prep for the week ahead.

   - Cook in bulk; freeze or store the extras.

   - Set up weekly menus to reduce decision fatigue.

- Serve easy "go-to" meals for days you feel worn out (like breakfast for dinner or soup).

- Tap into your gift of creativity and make mealtime fun by cooking together or making easy, kid-friendly meals (such as pancakes in the form of fun shapes).

- If financially feasible, order in on occasion.

- Put away the screens during mealtime.

2. **Sleep.** One of the most important aspects of sleep hygiene is consistent sleep and wake times. Here's how to help:

- As a family, decide each person's bedtime and then stick to it by using healthy boundaries set by parents and older children who are in charge of their own bedtime.

- Make sure everyone has a consistent bedtime routine (which should include soothing activities that support the transition to sleep).

- Set an alarm for when to start bedtime routines.

3. **Calendars.** To make the most of family calendars:

- Put all activities on a calendar that's accessible to everyone.

- If your children are old enough, teach them how to add their own schedules.

- Create a system if you need to be alerted about an event. For example, invite your partner as a "guest" on your virtual calendar to any events they need to be mindful of.

- If you prefer a physical calendar, options include a dry erase calendar, chalkboard, or more detailed, ADHD-friendly calendars available for purchase.

4. **School.** Here are ways to provide structure:

   - Prepare clothes, lunch, and backpack the night before. Encouraging children to participate in this can help empower them and build self-confidence.

   - Set a specific time for homework in a quiet, distraction-free setting. To avoid mismanagement of time, the earlier in the evening the better.

   - For younger children doing homework, set them up where they can be monitored and assisted.

   - If they have ADHD, investigate their eligibility for an IEP or 504 plan, which allows for accommodations such as homework being done during school hours.

   - Look into a tutor if needed. Some kids respond better to a person other than their parents.

   - Look into free online programs such as Schoolhouse.world. Many schools also offer online websites for extra practice in core subjects.

5. **Healthcare.** Follow these steps to streamline your family's healthcare needs:

   - Schedule appointments in advance for the entire year and mark all calendars.

   - Schedule all your children's appointments on the same day.

   - With prescriptions, acquire as many months at once as possible and try to coordinate pickups for the family on the same day.

   - Keep medications somewhere highly visible (but safe!) and stacked with another habit, such as brushing teeth.

- If remembering medication is an issue, set an alarm or purchase an alarm pill box.

6. **Rest time.** Whether your children are of napping age or not, their brains benefit from approximately 90 to 120 minutes of unstructured play or rest per day. As a family, choose a time that works for you. Most families fall into a natural rhythm with rest time.

7. **"Me" time.** As much as your children need rest time and unstructured play, to enhance your gift of energy, so do you. Review your Anti-Burnout Plan (page 124), then choose at least one self-care skill to do each day. It's also beneficial for your kids to see you prioritize and model self-care.

8. **Marriage/relationship.** Tending to your relationship can make working as a team easier. Schedule at least one date night a month (either in the home or out if possible), as well as one night per week to check in with one another. Time together makes a big difference for the entire family.

9. **Housework.** Even the youngest children can contribute with simple assigned chores or keeping their own room and toys picked up. For older children, this is a chance for them to learn household skills for their own future. Remember that enlisting others to contribute is a sign that you are instilling responsibility in others and avoiding burnout.

10. **Communication.** Keep reminders on dry erase boards or Boogie Board writing tablets around the house to help your family stay on track. When they complete a task, they can erase it. Another valuable communication device to consider is a free tracking app such as Life360, which tracks each family member's location and promotes peace of mind and safety.

Chapter Conclusion

While this chapter explored how to navigate pressures and expectations around parenting, the skills presented are useful for navigating all types of helpful relationships that women with ADHD find themselves in. Compassion fatigue and caretaker burnout can make managing ADHD difficult if you're not prioritizing your own needs. The many gifts and strengths of ADHD can benefit those you care for, but being the best you can be for others and yourself requires you to put yourself at the top of your priority list. Revisit the many self-care practices explored in this chapter any time you notice signs of burnout or overwhelm.

Chapter 11

Self-Care

Self-care is absolutely essential to your overall health and ability to be powered by your ADHD. Self-care is not indulgent; rather, it is a form of treatment and self-preservation. There are many reasons people with ADHD struggle with self-care, including unnecessary guilt, difficulty sustaining goals, lack of a role model, and life stress. Whatever the barrier, caring for yourself is a powerful way to improve your wellness and manage ADHD for the rest of your life.

MINDFULNESS

I recently met with a client with ADHD who was exploring her anxiety around not feeling present with her young children. She explored her fear of forgetting things, and came to realize while she was doing everything that she could to preserve memories (photographing, scrapbooking, etc.), the anxiety of forgetting was preventing her from being fully present and enjoying those moments.

It can be difficult for anyone, let alone a woman with ADHD, to quiet the racing thoughts and internal dialogue that interferes with noticing what is happening around them. This lack of presence can become detrimental in relationships. The tendency to feel distracted, interrupt, or forget things is common with ADHD, likely due to symptoms around impulse control, attention selection, and poor working memory.

Focus Meditation

In this exercise you'll practice a form of mindfulness meditation that can help improve your ability to be present, feel more engaged when socializing, and reduce potential issues with distractions or interruptions. To improve mindfulness, the goal is to integrate this or other meditations, as often as possible, as a foundation to the other self-care skills explored later in this chapter. Finally, if you prefer, you can find the recording of this meditation on my website at ameliakelley.com under "Book Resources." You may also choose to record yourself reading the instructions for this meditation, so you can follow along with the recording.

WHAT YOU WILL LEARN
- How ADHD is positively impacted by meditation
- How to use meditation to improve executive functioning and feel powered by ADHD

WHAT YOU WILL NEED (IN ADDITION TO TIME)
- A timer
- A quiet space to meditate

ADHD STRENGTHS
CREATIVITY, HYPERFOCUS

Instructions

1. Begin by finding a comfortable position to sit or lie down. Close your eyes or find an image or object to focus a soft gaze on.

2. Bring awareness to your body and feel the ground and air around you. Take a deep breath.

3. Relax your body, starting at the top of your head. Work your way down, relaxing your cheeks, jaw, neck, shoulders, back, stomach, hips, tops and bottoms of your legs, ankles, feet, and then toes.

4. Now focus your attention solely on your breath. Recite the words "in" on your inhale and "out" on your exhale for the next five cycles.

5. During this practice, your mind will likely wander. The challenge is not to empty your mind and achieve perfection, but rather practice *noticing* thinking and *noticing* your mind wandering.

6. When you notice your mind wander, recite the words "come back," and imagine bringing your focus to the center of your forehead.

7. At the completion of five cycles, return to your natural rhythm of breath.

8. Next, bring awareness to your breathing by counting each inhale and exhale cycle until you reach 10.

9. Return to your natural breathing.

10. Notice how your body feels in the space around you.

11. If you like, place your hands on your heart and bow your head in gratitude for taking the time to practice focus and self-love.

CONSIDERATIONS FOR A MEDITATION PRACTICE

Meditation can take on many forms, some of which work better for ADHD, especially when they involve anchor points for focus. You can even choose a mundane chore as a place to begin practicing; for example, mindfully washing the dishes, by noticing the feeling of the water on your skin, the weight of a glass in your hand, and the smell of the dish soap. Due to your ability to hyperfocus and your creative ADHD brain, you are more capable of immersing yourself in these tasks, and even a simple practice like this can help you build habits of intentional mindfulness.

Other options include:

- Progressive muscle relaxation

- Finding an image to focus on

- Guided meditations through apps such as Headspace or Insight Timer

- Recordings of binaural beats to increase concentration

- Counting or breath exercises

- Meditation groups

WALKING MEDITATION

If you find it difficult to meditate, try a walking meditation, which reduces the feeling of restlessness in the mind and body while trying to meditate.

1. Find a comfortable space where you can walk for at least 10 minutes without stopping.

2. Set a walking pace in which your body can remain calm.

3. Notice how your legs feel when you lift them up and forward and when your feet make contact with the ground.

4. Notice the sensation of your breath.

5. Take note of any other sensations you feel while walking.

6. As you walk, your mind may start to wander. Use the sounds around you and feelings of your steps and breathing to refocus your attention on the present.

7. If you like, look for guided walking meditations on Insight Timer and YouTube.

Whichever way you choose, the most important thing is consistency. Over time, meditation can help you become more mindful in your daily tasks and interactions. It can also center you, organize your thoughts and improve your executive functioning. Even if you only have one minute to meditate, it's far better than none.

TOP 5 MINDFULNESS TIPS TO CONTROL INTERRUPTING WITH ADHD

If you find interrupting is a common issue for you, mindfulness can help with this, too. Try these five mindfulness strategies:

1. **Breathe.** One common reason that interruptions occur is stress. Remember the breathing exercises that you practice in meditation and use them when in conversation. If you notice yourself becoming excited and engaged in a topic, remember to continue to breathe. Try a slow breath in and out to reset.

2. **Take notes.** You may fear forgetting an important point, so try jotting your thoughts down as they come to help relax and ground you. When it's your turn to speak, you may find the original thought no longer applies or, conversely, enhances the conversation.

3. **Repair when possible.** If you accidentally interrupt, keep it short. Acknowledge that you interrupted and encourage the person to continue talking. This acknowledgment can be validating for the other person and supports authentic connection.

4. **Prepare your body.** If you know you'll be in a situation where sustained attention is necessary, make sure you are well rested, exercise before the event, and if necessary, use a fidget or other soothing way to ground yourself. Even as a therapist, I use the cap of my water bottle, a pen, or dough to fidget with during sessions if I'm feeling physically or mentally drained.

5. **Ask permission.** Since working memory can be problematic for those with ADHD, if you have something you really want to share, you may try asking the other person if you can interject. This action is an interruption, but when done compassionately and framed as an effort to unmask your symptom of needing to remember your thought, it can help enhance intimacy and rapport.

SLEEP

One of the most effective forms of self-care is sleep. However, for women with ADHD, frustration about going to bed too late and struggling to fall asleep and stay asleep are common issues. This is because segmented sleep is common with ADHD, which on a neurological level, makes people with ADHD more alert to danger in the night.

Unfortunately, society demands we be monophasic sleepers (a sleep pattern occurring only once in 24 hours and most often at night) as opposed to biphasic sleep (where we sleep in two segments per day by napping) which the ADHD brain often finds more natural. Essentially, ADHD is responsible for some of our modern sleep issues, leaving many ADHD women feeling stuck despite their best efforts.

Thankfully, we are learning more about the connection between ADHD and sleep issues and how to improve it.

ADHD Sleep Plan

We'll explore the most common issues causing sleep disturbance for women with ADHD and what to do about it. With knowledge gathered from this section, you'll create your own sleep plan so you can finally get the sleep you need to feel your best.

Instructions

YOUR INTERNAL CLOCK

Many people with ADHD suffer from delayed sleep phase syndrome, characterized by the inability to fall asleep, difficulty waking up on time, and, in some cases, daytime sleepiness or depression. Over half of adults with ADHD report signs of this syndrome, and as a result many consider themselves to be "night owls" due to a very important mechanism in their brains being dysregulated; that is, their circadian rhythm, or internal clock.

While we all have natural circadian rhythms, there are differences in those with ADHD, who are more sensitive to the effects of light and stimulation. Women with ADHD may not always honor these natural rhythms and instead find themselves pushing past their natural sleep window, becoming overstimulated and hormonally stressed, causing insomnia and restlessness.

WHAT YOU WILL LEARN

- How ADHD impacts sleep quality
- Ways to overcome these challenges using effective sleep hygiene tailored specifically for those with ADHD

WHAT YOU WILL NEED (IN ADDITION TO TIME)

- A writing utensil
- This book or a journal

ADHD STRENGTH CREATIVITY

STIMULANTS

The ADHD brain craves stimulation. As a result, you may engage in stimulating activities right before bed, but this does not ease the mind into sleep. Similarly, women with ADHD who are managing career, home, and family may find they are medicating with caffeine. The rule of thumb is to discontinue drinking caffeinated beverages at least six hours before bed, as caffeine can take up to 10 hours to leave your system.

Many women with ADHD are also prescribed stimulant medication that can have a dramatic impact on sleep quality. If it seems like your medication is interfering with sleep, options include:

- Split dosing when possible (ask your doctor).

- Take your medication earlier in the day.

- Set your alarm 30 minutes before you need to get up, take your dose, and go back to sleep with a second alarm set for 30 minutes later.

- Talk to your doctor about trying non-stimulant, norepinephrine medications.

- Try a delayed-onset ADHD medication such as Jornay PM, which is taken at night. It takes about 10 hours to take effect and has the potential to alleviate issues with waking. (Note: There is no generic brand for this medication, so it may still be expensive.)

LIGHT

Melatonin is a hormone that's regulated by the sun and plays a large role in our ability to sleep. Research has found that those with ADHD tend to have a delay in natural melatonin production, being 90 minutes later than neurotypical brains. To address this, here are some recommendations:

- Take melatonin (under the tongue) 30 minutes to an hour before bed. Start with a minimal dose of 1 to 3 mg. Talk to a doctor about dosage and possible long-term effects, including a reduction in melatonin production and depressive symptoms.

- Light therapy is considered the best way to regulate our circadian rhythm and melatonin. Get out in the sun for at least 20 minutes as soon as possible upon waking. You can also use a full-spectrum light therapy lamp for at least 30 minutes a day, in addition to the 20 minutes of sunlight.

- Dim lights and limit screen time the hour before you go to bed. This helps protect you from potentially stimulating content as well as blue light that interferes with healthy melatonin production.

BEDTIME ROUTINE

Children aren't the only ones who need a bedtime routine! Adults do too, especially those with ADHD. One of the most important guidelines is to adhere to the same sleep and wake times, even on weekends. Any variation can throw off the delicate balance of your internal clock. To remedy this, you can try this relaxing and consistent bedtime routine:

- At least one hour before bedtime, reduce stimulation as much as possible—especially screens. If you can't resist these outlets, choose less stimulating options, such as some inspirational programming instead of the news.

- Enlist relaxing activities such as reading, taking a warm bath, talking with your partner in bed, crossword puzzles, meditating, or yoga.

- Tap into your creativity by creating art in a journal before bed. Interestingly, the areas of our brain that are most creative are more active during sleep, hence our tangential dreams, so your strength of creativity can be used to help encourage sleep when necessary.

- Listen to something relaxing, like YouTube recordings of Delta waves—low, deep waves that dominate your brain during deep, restorative sleep. Another option is hypnotherapist Thomas Hall's YouTube channel, with sleep and brainwave recordings to help induce sleep. (He also offers subliminal messaging recordings to help improve focus, attention, self-esteem and confidence.)

- If you suffer from restlessness or restless leg syndrome—which is common for those with ADHD—you may be transitioning too quickly into sleep. Try dimming the lights and gradually reducing activity at bedtime. Use a fan, noise machine, or soothing sounds to help you relax.

Based on what you've learned, establish your ADHD Sleep Plan to begin implementing tonight.

One hour before bed I will:

_____

_____

_____

_____

My plan for my medication, stimulants, or supplements includes:

_____

_____

_____

_____

I will support my transition from stimulation to sleep by:

_____

_____

_____

_____

My preferred sleep and wake times are:

_____

_____

_____

_____

Problematic behaviors that are not helping my sleep include:

_____

_____

_____

_____

I will change these behaviors by:

_____

_____

_____

_____

EXERCISE

What's your current relationship with exercise? You may be thinking, *I'm too busy, I used to exercise,* or *I just don't have it in me.* Many women with ADHD are so busy getting through their day that exercise doesn't happen. However, a lack of regular movement exacerbates ADHD symptoms. Conversely, exercise is a game changer for improving ADHD symptoms. Among other benefits, exercise:

- Improves focus and ability to concentrate

- Improves sleep

- Positively impacts executive functioning

- Changes the chemistry and circuitry in the brain in ways that provide both short- and long-term benefits

- Generates endorphins that help relieve pain, reduce stress, and increase your sense of well-being

While there are many short-term benefits to exercise, a long-term benefit includes an increase in a specific protein called **brain-derived neurotrophic factor**—or BDNF for short—found in high quantities in the brain. This protein plays a key role in the creation of new brain cells, and helps increase neuroplasticity, which helps us learn and remember new information. What this means is that, if you keep up with the habit of exercise, it can lead to growth in your brain. Exercise truly is more than just about how we look; it's an important form of mental and physical medicine.

ADHD Exercise Plan

The following exercise includes a step-by-step guide on how to overcome common barriers for starting and maintaining an exercise routine with ADHD. Strategies offered will highlight the strengths of while problem-solving potential barriers that result from executive functioning issues that cause women with ADHD to put self-care on the back burner. To conclude, a writing prompt will invite you to explore your reasons for prioritizing exercise as an additional motivational tool.

WHAT YOU WILL LEARN

- How to start and maintain an ADHD-friendly exercise routine
- Tricks for overcoming barriers to success

WHAT YOU WILL NEED (IN ADDITION TO TIME)

- A writing utensil
- A calendar for tracking

ADHD STRENGTHS
ENERGY, SPONTANEITY, HYPERFOCUS

Instructions

Start slow. Going all-in on exercise can lead to unrealistic expectations or injury. Instead, choose a minimal goal you believe you can succeed at. If you are not exercising at all, aiming to work out five days a week for 30 minutes may be excessive. Instead, you can set a goal for, say, 20 minutes two days a week. Once you succeed at that initial goal a few times, use your gift of energy and hyperfocus to set new ones until you reach your ultimate desired goal. Meeting goals feels good and encourages you to stick to your plan, while also reinforcing beliefs and neural networks around success that can help rewrite your narrative around exercise and goal-setting.

Seek accountability. Tracking how often you exercise is one way to remain accountable and receive consistent feedback about whether you exercised or not. Keep a simple calendar where you put a check mark when you worked out, and leave it blank when you didn't. Other options are having an accountability buddy to work out with or signing up for ADHD-friendly fitness coaching through websites like mycopilot. com. As you track the days you didn't work out, investigate what barriers made you miss that day. Remain compassionate with yourself—the more curious and inquisitive you remain, the more likely you will find solutions to things blocking your success.

Schedule efficiently. Until exercise becomes so habitual you no longer think about it, you will likely need a reminder. If you choose not to exercise, move the event to another time on your calendar, preferably later in that day. If you don't have as much time as you wanted, remember every little bit counts. While 30 minutes daily is ideal, even five minutes of movement is beneficial for jump-starting the secretion of healthy hormones and neurotransmitters that manage ADHD and well-being.

Reward yourself. Rewards matter to the ADHD brain! Especially because so much of a woman with ADHD's life can feel like work, it can be fun and enjoyable to receive instantaneous feedback for a job well done. Perhaps set a goal that, after five days of physical movement or exercise, you schedule self-care. Or perhaps the reward could be even more instantaneous; for instance, once you finish exercising, you take time to watch a movie or play a game.

Mix things up. The ADHD brain thrives off spontaneity and variety to help curb boredom. Instead of always running on a treadmill, switch things up and do something else that piques your interest and moves your body—tidying your home, gardening, walking to the store, playing a physical video game like on Nintendo Wii, dancing, or whatever you like. List ideas on your calendar so you have options.

Make it easy. If you need to drive all the way home from work to get your workout clothes and then head back to the gym, it's far less likely you will do it. Set up visual cues to remind you of your exercise goal and make it easy to get started. I keep hand weights in my office to encourage me to do short workouts in between client sessions if I don't have time to exercise at another point in the day. Every little bit counts.

SELF-COMPASSION MOTIVATION LETTER

Grab some notebook paper and write down what your hopes are for your exercise goal, as well as why it matters to you. You can also express any worries or concerns you may have about succeeding and how you plan to manage them. Make a copy of this letter and keep it somewhere that you can look at it if you get off track. You may also create a similar letter for other self-care goals you are creating while becoming powered by your ADHD.

WOMEN, HORMONES, AND ADHD

A woman's hormones, generally meant to help women bear children, can make ADHD management challenging. The female sex hormones, estrogen and progesterone, play a role in the severity of ADHD symptoms, and impact how well medication works.

Starting at puberty, a girl is flooded by a rapid increase in both estrogen and progesterone, which can cause symptoms such as depression, anxiety, impulsivity, and irritability, making ADHD symptoms harder to manage. Adding to this dramatic change, adolescent girls sometimes metabolize their medication more quickly, rendering it less effective.

The cycle continues into adulthood, as estrogen and progesterone levels continue to rise and fall over roughly 28 days. In the first two weeks of a woman's cycle (beginning with the onset of the period), they have the highest level of estrogen, making their mood brighter and ADHD symptoms appear more manageable. However, after ovulation, these levels drop as progesterone levels rise, making symptoms more difficult to manage until menstruation, when the cycle starts all over again.

The fun doesn't stop here! Typically in their forties, women enter perimenopause, when estrogen and progesterone levels become erratic and continue to drop about 65 percent over the next 10 years. The result is a drop in serotonin, dopamine, and norepinephrine, increasing sadness, irritability, fatigue, fuzzy thinking, memory lapses, and issues with inattention. These issues are prevalent even in women without ADHD, which is why perimenopause can be even more difficult for those who have the diagnosis.

Twelve months after a woman's last period, she enters menopause, and estrogen levels drop even further as does the trifecta of feel-good neurotransmitters. This drop can increase ADHD symptoms and have an effect on mood yet again. The good news, however, is that progesterone eventually becomes obsolete, which allows what estrogen there is left to become more effective at improving moods and making symptoms more manageable.

Taming the Hormone Roller Coaster

This strategy will enable you to make hormonal transitions and changes more manageable. You will learn how both medical and holistic approaches as well as everyday tools and tracking options will help you feel more in charge when your hormones go haywire.

Instructions

Find a tracker. One of the most effective strategies for navigating changing hormones is tracking. A tracking app like MyFLO can also clue you into possible hormone imbalances and suggest lifestyle changes (like the best foods to eat or activities to engage in) to feel better during different phases of your cycle. Knowing more about what you are going through and understanding why changes are happening allows for more balance and control. It also allows you to be gentle with yourself on days when your symptoms are less manageable.

Exercise. While some of us might be tempted to curl up on the couch when we're feeling crampy, fatigued, or uncomfortable, what we actually need is movement and hydration. It is helpful to maintain a gentle routine such as yoga, swimming, or walking when you have less energy, in addition to a regular workout routine for when you are feeling energized.

Use food as medicine. What you eat impacts your changing hormones as well as your mood, executive functioning, and other ADHD symptoms. Cutting

WHAT YOU WILL LEARN

- Effective ways to navigate hormonal changes and manage ADHD symptoms

WHAT YOU WILL NEED (IN ADDITION TO TIME)

- Access to a period tracker app (like MyFLO)

down on sugars and eating whole, unprocessed, nutrient-rich foods can help. Pay attention to how certain foods make you feel, and perhaps keep a food diary to see if certain foods intensify your symptoms.

Some foods that help improve symptoms include:

- Green tea
- Blueberries
- Red grapes
- Olive oil
- Organic or fermented soy
- Dark chocolate
- Turmeric
- Fatty fish
- Eggs
- Coffee

According to the National Institutes of Health, our gut provides approximately 95 percent of the body's serotonin, a key neurotransmitter needed to reduce issues of hyperactivity and impulsivity. By focusing on foods that your gut flora comprehends how to digest, you ensure that your brain is receiving more of the essential neurotransmitters it needs.

Look into hormone replacement. Especially during perimenopause and menopause, it can be helpful to talk with your doctor about hormone replacement therapy and, if necessary, antidepressants, if your mood is aggravating your ADHD symptoms. Studies have shown that hormone replacement therapy helps ADHD treatment and medications work more effectively. There are also several holistic herbs hitting the market that can help balance women's hormones during perimenopause and menopause.

Explore herbal remedies. Whether you are on ADHD medication or not, it can be helpful to explore the possibility of using vitamins, minerals, and other herbal supplements to support your hormonal fluctuations as well as overall management of ADHD. Always check with a medical provider before starting any herbal regimen. A functional (holistic) doctor or a traditional medical provider well-versed in ADHD can assess for issues such as low vitamin D levels, adrenal fatigue, and gut health. Some issues they may address would include:

ISSUE	REMEDY
Distractibility	Vitamin D (with K2 for absorption)
Brain fog	Probiotics/pancreatic enzymes
Focus	Tyrosine
Depression	L-tryptophan/5-HTP
Anxiety	L-theanine
Mood swings	Check hormone levels/DHEA

Chapter Conclusion

Self-care is an absolute necessity. This is true for everyone, and especially women with ADHD. While self-care can be challenging to prioritize with the responsibilities of everyday life, it does not need to be extravagant or time-consuming.

Some forms of self-care are free, such as deep breathing, taking a warm bath, going for a walk, talking to a friend, getting to sleep on time, or setting necessary boundaries. Play, which adults do not do enough of, is also important, as is learning something new or doing a hobby you love.

Other forms of self-care can be more challenging, such as therapy or self-help, which require us to confront things that aren't necessarily working for us. Whichever forms of self-care you choose, make sure to get the most out of every moment.

Chapter Twelve

Relationships

ADHD can have a significant impact on relationships. Misunderstandings and resentment in close relationships around things like boredom, distractibility, bluntness, interruptions, forgetfulness, and inattention are some of the more common issues. There are, however, very effective ways to build healthier and happier relationships. The following chapter explores common pitfalls that occur in many ADHD relationships as well as specific skills and mindset shifts that can lead to happier, healthier relationships.

INTIMACY

One of my clients with ADHD recently expressed anxiety about whether the relationship she was in was the right one. Up until this point, everything she shared about their relationship was very positive and hopeful. Her concern appeared to stem from a common issue that arises for people with ADHD: boredom.

According to a 2015 NYU study, the honeymoon stage typically lasts anywhere from three to six months, which coincides with the reduction in excess dopamine that floods our brains early on in dating. Considering that people with ADHD don't have as many dopamine receptors, they respond well to the excess dopamine delivered to the brain when falling for someone. This also means they more acutely feel when the honeymoon phase is ending, though they may not realize that it could cause them to disengage.

Unfortunately, if efforts are not made to reconnect in a healthy way, you may find yourself sabotaging a relationship to increase intensity and reward to the ADHD brain. Other potential issues include cheating or breaking up without significant reasons, or chronically dating new people to feel the sense of excitement.

Sustaining Connection

We'll explore the top three motivators the ADHD brain receives in the beginning stages of a relationship, and how these motivators can be sustained long-term. Exploring these needs with your partner will help improve intimacy, enhance engagement, and offer opportunities to reclaim excitement in your relationship.

WHAT YOU WILL LEARN

- The importance of novelty and healthy challenges for women with ADHD
- How to achieve these needs with your partner to improve your relationship's health

ADHD STRENGTHS
CREATIVITY, SPONTANEITY, HYPERFOCUS

Instructions

TOP 3 MOTIVATORS FOR ADHD RELATIONSHIPS

1. **Interest or passion.** The chemical dopamine (closely associated with our brain's reward centers) increases dramatically when we are falling in love. Meanwhile, the stress hormone cortisol also rises, which subsequently reduces serotonin. Low levels of serotonin cause intrusive thoughts, such as preoccupations and obsessions—in this case, the infatuation of new love. This is why the early stages of love can make people with ADHD hyperfocused on their new love interest.

2. **Challenge.** The chase and success of being with the person you want can be exhilarating. Even if it was an easy catch, chemicals ignite the reward centers of the brain, producing responses that can rival the exhilaration of overcoming the greatest challenges—a speeding heart, sweaty palms, flushed cheeks, and even anxiety. There's also the

challenge of getting to know the other person and the uncertainty as to whether this new connection will grow.

3. **Novelty.** It's easy to see how the need for novelty is satisfied early in a relationship. Many people feel they "never run out of things to talk about." Even mundane tasks such as grocery shopping can feel romantic. For some, falling in love exposes them to feelings and parts of themselves they never knew existed. The novelty of a new relationship is potent in keeping the attention of someone with ADHD.

HOW TO MAINTAIN INTIMACY WITH THESE MOTIVATORS

1. **Interest or passion.** As a relationship stabilizes, the roller coaster of hormones, emotions, and neurotransmitters returns to normal levels and the stress of new love is gone. For those with ADHD, the drop in dopamine can lead to feelings of boredom, distractibility, and consciously or unconsciously pulling away.

   The research provides hope, however. According to a study at Stony Brook University, even those in long-term relationships still have the same intensity of activation in dopamine-rich areas of the brain as those who are newly in love. This suggests that the excitement of romance can remain while the stress of new love is lost.

   How exactly, then, do you reconnect with these reward systems and reinvigorate passion?

   • Prioritize sexual activity and physical intimacy, such as giving a massage, sitting close, napping together, or holding hands. The research highlighted physical touch and other forms of intimacy as the reason these reward centers remained active. Pay attention to when your gift of energy is at its highest and aim for closeness and connect during those times.

- Have open conversations about how often each partner desires connection, whether it be physical or otherwise.

- If feeling too overwhelmed for physical intimacy, do things that relax your body first so you feel more available to your partner.

2. **Challenge.** For the ADHD brain that thrives on spontaneity and challenge, it's important to continue seeking different ways to challenge one another. The most effective way to do this? Practice open authenticity and curiosity.

   Relationships offer challenges—we only miss out on them when we don't openly discuss them. If you feel short on inspiration sitting at home, take your conversation elsewhere, and use your surroundings as a springboard for authentic discussion. Relationship intimacy games such as the BestSelf Co. Intimacy Deck can also help spark connection and deeper conversation.

   Whether it be game night, reading books to discuss with each other, asking the hard questions, practicing spirituality together, or learning more through couples' counseling, connecting authentically offers meaningful challenges that can keep passion alive.

3. **Novelty.** As relationships shift toward compassionate, stable, and lasting love, it also becomes familiar and can start to feel old and worn. But you can still experience novelty as a couple.

   Major life transitions are one way novelty manifests in long-term relationships. Parenting, moving into a new home, starting a new job, or dealing with a loss can all be stressful but also thrust the relationship back into a space of novelty.

   You can also create healthy ways to experience novelty together. If your gift of spontaneity has inspired you to try something new, maybe try including your partner. It can even feed the need for challenge, with some healthy competition between one another, creating the passion you seek.

AUTHENTICITY AND RELATIONSHIP ACCOMMODATIONS

One of the most important ways to maintain a healthy, intimate relationship with ADHD is authenticity. Asking for what you need allows for open conversation about potential relationship accommodations, which are reasonable adjustments made to meet one another's needs. While being overly accommodating can lead to codependency patterns (a tendency to do more than your share in a relationship, especially to the detriment of your well-being), most healthy relationships involve compromise. Common examples of relationship accommodations for ADHD include:

- Taking on mundane tasks that take prolonged focus for the partner with ADHD

- Reminding the ADHD partner about tasks, appointments, or events

- Splitting roles so each person does what they're best at

- Working to not build resentment with one another

- Empathizing with one another

- Understanding the impact of hormones on ADHD symptoms

- Being mindful of the other's social needs, wishes, and limitations

- Changing routines as needed and working together to create them

- Prioritizing finances and resources for treatment or other supportive services

It's important to check in with each other and have open and honest conversations about how ADHD impacts each partner and what each partner can do to offer support.

MASKING IN RELATIONSHIPS

Masking, as we explored briefly in the section on ADHD trauma, happens when someone makes personal changes to cover up or compensate for symptoms. Masking is a way to fit societal norms through avoiding behaviors that naturally make people with ADHD feel comfortable. A person who is masking, for instance, may work to keep their fidgeting within the norm, and avoid the kinds of bouncing or rocking motions that would comfort them but be much more noticeable.

While some masking behaviors can help, such as writing things down to remember them, there can be negative effects of masking, including:

- Ignoring self-care and personal needs

- Struggling to fit in

- Feeling burnt out

- Struggling with imposter's syndrome, which affects self-confidence

- Mental health issues, such as anxiety or depression from constantly feeling under stress

- Barriers to proper diagnosis and treatment due to masking

The more you mask, the less connection you have with your authentic needs, and the more difficult it becomes to connect with others. Thankfully, you can find success with ADHD in a neurotypical world while also releasing the pressure of masking.

Unmasking ADHD

Learn about yourself in this self-assessment of commonly used ADHD masking behaviors and reflect on how ones you use might be affecting your life and relationships. From there, you'll learn specific coping skills for unmasking ADHD in a way that still provides a sense of safety and control. Finally, you'll have the chance to engage in a five-minute "unmasking meditation."

Instructions

Read the common masking behaviors that women with ADHD use to minimize symptoms in social settings. Check off any that have applied to you in the past as well as currently.

Making excuses for being late
— Past   — Present

Not admitting you missed information if distracted
— Past   — Present

Putting in substantially more effort and time than others to achieve a goal
— Past   — Present

Pressuring yourself to complete tasks before a deadline
— Past   — Present

Ignoring self-care needs to meet deadlines
— Past   — Present

WHAT YOU WILL LEARN
- How to identify harmful masking behaviors
- How you can respond with mindfulness, authenticity, and self-acceptance

WHAT YOU WILL NEED (IN ADDITION TO TIME)
- A writing utensil
- This book or a journal
- A quiet space

**ADHD STRENGTH
CREATIVITY**

Checking your work multiple times before submitting

—— Past   —— Present

Obsessively checking your belongings to make sure you haven't lost them

—— Past   —— Present

Focusing intensely during conversations to keep up

—— Past   —— Present

Being extra early to events to avoid being late

—— Past   —— Present

Hiding the use of alarms and reminders

—— Past   —— Present

Writing things down even in the middle of a conversation

—— Past   —— Present

Excessive fatigue

—— Past   —— Present

Feeling disconnected from who you are

—— Past   —— Present

Exhibiting perfectionistic tendencies

—— Past   —— Present

Mimicking or copying other people in social situations

—— Past   —— Present

Reacting as you believe people expect you to

—— Past   —— Present

Suppressing stimulating behaviors like leg bouncing

—— Past   —— Present

Remaining quiet or overly careful about what you say

—— Past   —— Present

For any masking behaviors you only did in the past, even as a child, journal in the space below about how you let go of these masking behaviors:

_____

_____

_____

_____

_____

By being open and unmasking, you allow your friends and family to better understand you and how to best support you. Unmasking also helps alleviate emotional pressure and exhaustion caused by suppressing how you feel when trying to fit in. While recognizing masking is the first step, there are additional ways to unmask your ADHD and feel more empowered in doing so.

FOUR TIPS FOR UNMASKING ADHD

1. **Use accommodations.** After identifying your masking behaviors, explore accommodations or creative alternatives that help manage your symptoms. For example, if you feel the need to fidget, find a discreet fidget toy or even use the tip of your pen to keep your hands busy—anything that helps manage symptoms while allowing you to stay engaged. Likewise, if large gatherings drain you, make a point to leave before you feel the need to overcompensate with masking behaviors.

2. **Open up.** Identify people that you feel comfortable with to talk with about ADHD challenges. As you receive positive or neutral feedback on your self-expression, your confidence will grow.

3. **Unmask together.** When you open up to friends, family, or peers, they too may share their own experiences with masking in some way to compensate for some perceived social nonconformity. There are also in-person and virtual support groups where you can practice unmasking.

4. **Seek treatment.** ADHD treatments such as medication, coaches, and therapies are designed to help you manage the symptoms you're trying to mask. Through treatment, you can work to identify your strengths and reduce self-limiting beliefs. You will also be more likely to recognize when masking behaviors are hurting you rather than helping you.

UNMASKING ADHD MEDITATION

Use this meditation before engaging in interactions that normally increase your masking tendencies. You can find a recording of this meditation at ameliakelley.com on the "Book Resources" page.

1. Begin in a comfortable position, sitting or lying down. If you like, close your eyes.

2. Take a deep, slow breath into the base of your belly. Hold for the count of four, and then slowly release the breath to the count of six.

3. Return to normal breathing and notice the natural rise and fall of your breath as you settle into your body.

4. Let go of the idea that you are here to empty your mind. Simply notice any thoughts that arise.

5. In your mind, imagine a time when you were masking.

6. Recognize any experiences within your body when thinking of this, and notice where you feel the most tension.

7. This area of tension is your masking center—it signals to you when you are masking. Mindfully breathe into that space until you feel the tension release even slightly.

8. Bring your attention to the muscles in your face. Feel the air against your cheeks, forehead, nose, and chin, and give yourself permission to let go of the tension in all these spaces.

9. On your next inhale, breathe into your masking center, and on each exhale, imagine the muscles of your face becoming more relaxed. (If the masking center is also your face, imagine breathing into the center of your forehead.) Do this for at least five full cycles of breath in and out.

10. Come back to the instance where you originally imagined masking and see how the tension feels in your body now. If it still feels intense, repeat the previous breath pattern (steps 7 through 9).

11. Finally, bring your attention to your heart center, and if you like, place your hands over your heart.

12. As you inhale and exhale into your heart center, begin repeating the phrase (either out loud or in your mind) "I love and accept myself." Do this until you feel open to the message or soften to it.

13. Rest your hands in your lap and return to normal breathing. Scan your body for any tension, and breathe deeply into any spaces you need to further release.

14. Refocus on the space you are in. Notice the sounds, the light, and the feel of the air around you. When you are ready, gently open your eyes.

15. Take a moment to express gratitude to yourself for taking this time to unmask your ADHD.

RELATIONSHIP WITH SELF

As we've explored throughout this book, the way you feel about yourself and come to understand the gifts of your ADHD has a big impact on how well you can manage your symptoms. Self-compassion is at the forefront of making positive changes, because you are more likely to change when you feel supported, understood, and loved. If you meet your challenges with frustration and negative self-talk, your self-esteem and confidence will suffer, as will your relationship with yourself.

Ideally, getting to know yourself better includes gaining a sense of pride, ownership, and acceptance of the wonderful gifts your ADHD brain possesses. When we're feeling down on some part of ourselves, it's important to keep in mind that no part of us is inherently "bad"—all parts really just want the best for us. So, if you have a part of you that is avoiding responsibilities or making your life more difficult, it may help to ask that part what it needs. Oftentimes, the answer is "rest." If you can understand yourself and your experience, you'll be better able to use the strategies in this book to regulate yourself, unmask, and meet your own needs.

Compassionate Self-Talk

This final strategy will help you learn how to speak to yourself as a friend using the power of self-compassion and a growth mindset. Use your ADHD strength of creativity to think of new ways to speak to yourself with compassion. By identifying your ADHD struggles and noticing how you speak to yourself, you will find a more energizing and motivating way to meet your goals.

Instructions

Take a moment to reflect on some of the common ADHD challenges you have faced. Some ideas might include forgetfulness, distractibility, being late, and so forth. Write these struggles in the left column in the chart on page 171.

1. Once you fill out the first column, think about what you would normally say to yourself when feeling frustrated about each of those challenges. Write that in the next column.

2. After completing the second column, go back and read what you would say to yourself. Take a moment to imagine saying these things to a friend.

3. Connect with your body and notice how it feels. Recognize whether you feel motivated to take action for change after the way you normally speak to yourself.

WHAT YOU WILL LEARN

- The importance of self-compassion and positive self-talk to improve your relationship with yourself
- How to increase your positive perceptions about being a woman with ADHD

WHAT YOU WILL NEED (IN ADDITION TO TIME)

- A writing utensil
- This book or a journal

ADHD STRENGTH CREATIVITY

4. Next, fill out the last column by reacting to that same struggle as if you were speaking to a friend.

5. Connect again with your body and notice how it feels. Recognize whether you feel motivated to facilitate change after speaking with a more compassionate tone.

As you continue working toward self-compassion, pay attention to the speed and tone of your voice. Try the simple trick of slowing the pace of your speech and quieting your tone. A large portion of what we express is in our tone of voice and not even what we say; consequently, these shifts can soothe your nervous system and improve your ability to regulate your vagus nerve, which aids in body functions and the ability to feel safe.

Take a moment to journal about the experience and what you noticed:

_____

_____

_____

_____

_____

_____

_____

_____

_____

PERSONAL ADHD STRUGGLES	WHAT YOU WOULD NORMALLY SAY TO YOURSELF ABOUT THIS CHALLENGE.	HOW YOU WOULD SPEAK TO A FRIEND FACING THE SAME CHALLENGE.

Chapter Conclusion

After countless times experiencing disappointment, rejection, or shame, especially when it comes to relationships, it can feel difficult to believe in yourself. Throughout this book, we have explored how ADHD can enhance and enrich a woman's life as well as create challenges and barriers to what you want to achieve for yourself. One of the most important components to achieving what you desire is getting over the wall of doubt to the other side. ADHD coach Brendan Mahan suggests taking these four steps:

1. **Notice the wall.** By at least knowing it is there (doubt, fear, rejection sensitivity), this brings you to the present so you can forge ahead.
2. **Don't try to blast through it.** This can look like negative self-talk, white knuckling, criticism, self-bullying. While these approaches may have worked in the past, these tactics won't improve your self-esteem or relationship with yourself in the present.
3. **Don't avoid the wall by going around it, as it will still be standing there waiting for you next time.** This may look like avoidance tactics, procrastination, or ignoring how you feel altogether.
4. **Take your time and move mindfully through it.** He suggests putting a door in the wall, where you know you will go through when you are ready. Choose from the strategies in this book to form a door to move through when the timing is right. This practice is a gentler, more compassionate way to make changes. When you want to make a big change or overcome a wall of doubt, know that it's okay to process your feelings and reactions and come back when you're ready.

Remember that with every struggle comes a gift, and with every gift there might be challenges. Know that you are not meant to fit into anyone else's box, and as you continue to recreate yourself, you will fit into your own. Like every other aspect of life, there is no end to learning and growing when you fully love and accept yourself.

CONCLUSION

It is time for women with ADHD to stop doubting themselves, their abilities, and the unique strengths they have to offer. Being powered by ADHD means accepting the parts of ADHD that are most challenging and knowing that perfection is not the goal. Radical acceptance and appreciating all of who you are also does not mean getting "rid" of symptoms altogether. Instead, it means that, when you get off track, as we all do, you can choose self-love and self-compassion. Return often to the skills and techniques in this book that most resonated with you. The more you practice these skills, the more awareness you will have about yourself and your ADHD.

Going forward, I hope you'll choose to recognize and love your beautiful, unique, diverse, and highly skilled brain. Make daily efforts to release any shame you once felt about ADHD. Know that what makes you different from neurotypicals is what makes you extraordinary. Let go of the idea that fitting into boxes of "normalcy" is a good thing. These boxes are limiting and harmful and force young girls and women with ADHD or any neurodivergence to stop believing in themselves. When challenge arises, ask for what you need, as you deserve to be supported. And finally, remember that every single day there is an opportunity to use your ADHD gifts and strengths, allowing you to positively impact both your life and the world around you.

RESOURCES

Online Resources

ADDitude Magazine
www.additudemag.com
A comprehensive website of ADHD-related articles, webinars, and resources.

Fitness Blender
www.fitnessblender.com
Workouts, healthy recipes, relaxing meditations, and expert articles, for a whole body and mind approach to feeling great.

How to ADHD (YouTube)
www.youtube.com/@HowtoADHD
Friendly and shame-free advice on how to survive and even thrive in a world not always built for the ADHD brain. Hosted by writer and ADHD pioneer Jessica McCabe.

The Huberman Lab Podcast
www.hubermanlab.com/podcast
Distills complex topics into accessible advice on topics like ADHD, helping listeners hack the way the nervous system works to benefit well-being.

The Mel Robbins Podcast
www.melrobbins.com/podcast
Deeply personal stories, relatable topics, and tactical, research-backed advice to help you create a better life.

My CoPilot
www.mycopilot.com/ADHD
ADHD-friendly coaching to reach your health and fitness goals. Receive support from a live coach who personalizes a plan to keep you accountable, motivated, and on track.

TEDxKinjarling "ADHD in Girls and Women" (YouTube)

www.youtube.com/watch?v=ybk2IzwV6Zg

Martha Barnard-Rae explores living with undiagnosed ADHD for 39 years, and the reasons girls and women are underdiagnosed.

A Slob Comes Clean

www.aslobcomesclean.com

A safe place to know you are not alone in your housekeeping struggles, featuring host Dana K. White.

Books

ADHD: A Hunter in a Farmer's World (Third Edition) by Thom Hartman

A groundbreaking book that explains how people with ADHD are not disordered or dysfunctional but simply "hunters in a farmer's world," and offers concrete non-drug methods and practices to help embrace their differences, nurture creativity, and find success.

The ADHD Effect on Marriage: Understand and Rebuild Your Relationship in Six Steps by Melissa Orlov

An invaluable resource for couples in which one of the partners suffers from ADHD. Orlov offers advice from her own personal experience and years of research, helping readers identify and overcome patterns of behavior that can hurt their marriages.

Divergent Mind: Thriving in a World that Wasn't Designed For You by Jenera Nerenberg

Explores why neurodivergent traits are overlooked in women and how society benefits from allowing their unique strengths to flourish.

How to ADHD: An Insider's Guide to Working with Your Brain (Not Against It) by Jessica McCabe

An honest, friendly, and shame-free guide, written by the creator of the award-winning YouTube channel *How to ADHD*, in which she shares the hard-won insights and practical strategies that have helped her survive, even thrive, in a world not built for her brain.

Taking Charge of Adult ADHD: Proven Strategies to Succeed at Work, at Home, and in Relationships (Second Edition) by Russell A. Barkley
Explores what ADHD looks like in adults, how to get an accurate evaluation, and how sufferers can manage symptoms and build the life they want. Includes skill-building exercises plus clear answers to questions about medications and other treatments.

Women with Attention Deficit Disorder (Second Edition) by Sari Solden
Explores treatment and counseling options, and uses real-life case histories to examine the special challenges women with ADD and ADHD face.

REFERENCES

Part I

Armstrong, Thomas. "The Myth of the Normal Brain: Embracing Neurodiversity." *AMA Journal of Ethics* 17.4 (2015): 348–352.

Ashinoff, B.K., Abu-Akel, A. "Hyperfocus: the forgotten frontier of attention." *Psychological Research* 85, 1–19 (2021). https://doi.org/10.1007/s00426-019-01245-8

Barnard-Rae, Martha. "ADHD in Girls and Women." YouTube. Video, 16:36. https://www.youtube.com/watch?v=ybk2IzwV6Zg.

Baum, J. (2022). *Anxiously Attached: Becoming more secure in life and love.* Penguin Random House.

Belski, Gail. "The difference between ADHD and executive function challenges." Understood. Accessed on 6/20/2023. https://www.understood.org/en/articles/difference-between-executive-functioning-issues-and-adhd.

Chaplin, Tara M. "Gender and Emotion Expression: A Developmental Contextual Perspective." Emot Rev. 2015 Jan;7(1):14-21. doi: 10.1177/1754073914544408. PMID: 26089983; PMCID: PMC4469291.

Chayka, Kyle. "Playing Tetris Will Make You Forget You're Hungry." *Time.* March 6, 2014. https://time.com/14021/playing-tetris-will-make-you-forget-youre-hungry.

Croley, K.E., Drevon, D.D., Decker, D.M. et al. "The Effect of the Fidget Cube on Classroom Behavior among Students with Perceived Attention Difficulties." *Behavior Analysis in Practice* 16.2 (2023)/ 547-557.

Franken, R. (2007). *Human Motivation.* Thomas Wadsworth.

Gaub, Miranda, and Caryn L. Carlson. "Gender differences in ADHD: A meta-analysis and critical review." *Journal of the American Academy of Child & Adolescent Psychiatry* 36.8 (1997): 1036-1045.

Han, D.H., D. McDuff, D. Thompson, M.E. Hitchcock, C.L. Reardon, B. Hainline. "Attention-deficit/hyperactivity disorder in elite athletes: a narrative review." *Br J Sports Med.* 2019 Jun;53(12):741-745. doi: 10.1136/bjsports-2019-100713. Epub 2019 May 16. PMID: 31097459.

Hartman, T. (2019) *ADHD: A Hunter in a Farmer's World 3rd ed.* Inner Traditions/Bear and Company.

Healey, Dione M., and Julia J. Rucklidge. "The relationship between ADHD and creativity." *The ADHD Report* 16.3 (2008)/ 1-5.

Hinchcliffe, Emma. "Women CEOs run 10.4% of Fortune 500 companies. A quarter of the 52 leaders became CEO in the last year." *Fortune*. June 5, 2023. https://fortune.com/2023/06/05/fortune-500-companies-2023-women-10-percent.

Hupfeld, K.E., T.R. Abagis, P. Shah. "Living "in the zone": hyperfocus in adult ADHD." *Atten Defic Hyperact Disord*. 2019 Jun;11(2):191-208. doi: 10.1007/s12402-018-0272-y. Epub 2018 Sep 28. Erratum in: Atten Defic Hyperact Disord. 2019 Mar 8: PMID: 30267329.

Jackson, S.A. "Joy, Fun, and Flow State in Sport." In: Y.L. Hanin, Ed., Emotions in Sport, Human Kinetics Publishers, Champaign, 2000, pp. 135-155.

Jelinek, Michael S. "Don't Let ADHD Crush Children's Self-Esteem." *MDEdge*. May 1, 2010. https://www.mdedge.com/psychiatry/article/23971/pediatrics/dont-let-adhd-crush-childrens-self-esteem.

Jordan, Michele. "Adult ADHD: Statistics and Facts." WebMD. July 13, 2022. https://www.webmd.com/add-adhd/adult-adhd-facts-statistics.

Lapera, N. (2022) *How to Meet Your Self: The Workbook for Self-Discovery*. Harper Collins.

Liao, Sharon. "How to Use Hyperfocus for Good." WebMD.com. September 1, 2022. https://www.webmd.com/add-adhd/ss/slideshow-adhd-hyperfocus-tips.

Nazeer, A, M. Mansour, K.A. Gross. "ADHD and adolescent athletes." *Front Public Health*. 2014 Jun 17;2/46. doi/ 10.3389:fpubh.2014.00046. PMID/ 24987666; PMCID/ PMC4060024.

Price, Devon. *Unmasking Autism: Discovering the New Faces of Neurodiversity*. First Edition. New York, NY: Harmony Books, 2022.

Richards, Amanda. "'Working: What We Do All Day' Explores What a 'Good' Job Actually Is." Tudum by Netflix. May 17, 2023. https://www.netflix.com/tudum/articles/barack-obama-working-docuseries.

Runco, Mark A. *Divergent Thinking*. Norwood, NJ/ Ablex Publishing Corporation, 1991.

Sedgwick, Jane Ann, Andrew Merwood, and Philip Asherson. "The positive aspects of attention deficit hyperactivity disorder/ a qualitative investigation of successful adults with ADHD." *ADHD Attention Deficit and Hyperactivity Disorders*. 11 (2019)/ 241-253.

Skogli, Erik Winther, et al. "ADHD in girls and boys–gender differences in co-existing symptoms and executive function measures." *BMC psychiatry* 13.1 (2013): 1-12.

Steglich-Peterson, Asbjørn and Varga, Zomogy. "Curiosity and Zetetic Style in ADHD." Philarchive.org. Accessed on 6/28/2023. https://philarchive.org/archive/STECAZ.

Suttie, Jill. "How to Listen to Pain." *Greater Good*. February 17, 2016. https://greatergood.berkeley.edu/article/item/

how_to_listen_to_pain#:~:text=According%20to%20Bren%C3%A9%20
Brown%2C%20a,we%20interact%20in%20the%20world.

Understood. "Celebrity spotlight: Why journalist Lisa Ling was 'relieved' by her ADHD
diagnosis." Accessed on 6/1/2023. https://www.understood.org/en/articles/
celebrity-spotlight-why-journalist-lisa-ling-was-relieved-by-her-adhd-diagnosis.

White, Holly A. "Thinking "outside the box": Unconstrained creative generation in
adults with attention deficit hyperactivity disorder." *The Journal of Creative
Behavior* 54.2 (2020): 472-483.

Young, Jeffrey R. "Researcher Behind '10,000-Hour Rule' Says Good Teaching
Matters, Not Just Practice." EdSurge. May 5, 2020. https://www.edsurge.com/
news/2020-05-05-researcher-behind-10-000-hour-rule-says-good-teaching-
matters-not-just-practice.

Zoratto, Francesca, et al. "Methylphenidate administration promotes sociability and
reduces aggression in a mouse model of callousness." *Psychopharmacology*
236 (2019)/ 2593-2611.

Part II

Anderson, K.N. et. al. "ADHD Medication Use During Pregnancy and Risk for
Selected Birth Defects: National Birth Defects Prevention Study, 1998-2011."
Journal of Attention Disorders. 2020; 24 (3): 479-489.

Bangma, Dorien F. et al. "Financial decision-making in adults with ADHD."
Neuropsychology 33.8 (2019): 1065.

Beauchaine, Theodore P., Itzhak Ben-David, and Marieke Bos. "ADHD, financial
distress, and suicide in adulthood: A population study." *Science advances*
6.40 (2020): eaba1551.

Brannen, Julia, Rebecca O'Connell, and Ann Mooney. "Families, meals and
synchronicity: eating together in British dual earner families." *Community, Work
& Family* 16.4 (2013): 417-434.

BUMPS. "Methylphenidate." January 2023, Version 4. https://
www.medicinesinpregnancy.org/Medicine—pregnancy/
Methylphenidate/#:~:text=Some%20studies%20have%20suggested%20
that,not%20have%20a%20birth%20defect.

CDC. "Use of ADHD Medicine is Increasing among Pregnant Women." Accessed
on 6/15/2023. https://www.cdc.gov/pregnancy/meds/treatingfortwo/features/
keyfinding-ADHD-med-increase.html.

CHEMM. "FDA Pregnancy Categories."Accessed on 7/1/2023, 2024. https://chemm.
hhs.gov/pregnancycategories.htm.

Chun Wong, Heng, and Rashid Zaman. "Neurostimulation in treating ADHD."
Psychiatria Danubina 31.suppl 3 (2019): 265-275.

Clear, James. *Atomic Habits: Tiny Changes, Remarkable Results: An Easy & Proven Way to Build Good Habits & Break Bad Ones*. New York, NY. Avery, an imprint of Penguin Random House, 2018.

Cuddy, Amy J.C., Caroline Ashley Wilmuth, and Dana R. Carney. "The benefit of power posing before a high-stakes social evaluation." *Harvard Business School working paper series #13-027* (2012).

Dorani, F., D. Bijlenga, A. Beekman, E. van Someren, and J. Kooij. (2021). "Prevalence of hormone-related mood disorder symptoms in women with ADHD." *Journal of Psychiatric Research, 133*, 10–15. https://doi.org/10.1016/j.jpsychires.2020.12.005

Enright, Jillian. "ADHD Paralysis Explained." (2021): Retrieved May 22, 2023. https://original.newsbreak.com/@jillian-enright-1590470/2420107533437-adhd-paralysis-explained.

Finkel, E.J., W.K. Campbell. "Self-control and accommodation in close relationships: an interdependence analysis." *J Pers Soc Psychol*. 2001 Aug;81(2):263-77. doi: 10.1037//0022-3514.81.2.263. PMID: 11519931.

Gilligan, Chris. "How the Pandemic Boosted Working From Home." *U.S. News*. May 18, 2023. https://www.usnews.com/news/health-news/articles/2023-05-18/how-the-covid-pandemic-impacted-working-from-home.

Ginapp, Callie M., Norman R. Greenberg, Grace Macdonald-Gagnon, Gustavo A. Angarita, Krysten W. Bold, and Marc N. Potenza. "The experiences of adults with ADHD in interpersonal relationships and online communities: A qualitative study" *SSM—Qualitative Research in Health*, Volume 3, 2023,100223, ISSN 2667-3215, https://doi.org/10.1016/j.ssmqr.2023.100223

Gordon, Chanelle T., and Stephen P. Hinshaw. "Executive functions in girls with and without childhood ADHD followed through emerging adulthood: Developmental trajectories." *Journal of Clinical Child & Adolescent Psychology* (2019).

Hacking Your ADHD. "Important But Not Urgent (IBNU)." Podcast, 14:31. https://www.hackingyouradhd.com/podcast/important-but-not-urgent-ibnu.

Harrison, Yvonne and James A. Horne. "The impact of sleep deprivation on decision making: a review." *Journal of experimental psychology/ Applied 6.3* (2000)/ 236.

Justice, A.J., de Wit, H. (1999). "Acute Effects of D-Amphetamine During the Follicular and Luteal Phases of the Menstrual Cycle in Women." *Psychopharmacology (Berl)*. https://doi.org/10.1007/s002130051033.

Kelley, Amelia. "How the Neurodiverse Can Better Cope With Decision Fatigue." *Psychology Today*. July 17, 2023. https://www.psychologytoday.com/us/blog/in-your-corner/202307/neurodiversity-coping-with-decision-fatigue.

Klil-Drori, Sivan, and Lily Hechtman. "Potential social and neurocognitive benefits of aerobic exercise as adjunct treatment for patients with ADHD." *Journal of Attention Disorders* 24.5 (2020): 795-809.

Lee, Clara S.C. et al. "The effectiveness of mindfulness-based intervention in attention on individuals with ADHD: A systematic review." *Hong Kong Journal of Occupational Therapy* 30.1 (2017): 33-41.

Liao, Chi. "ADHD symptoms and financial distress." *Review of Finance* 25.4 (2021): 1129-1210.

Lorber, M.F., A.C. Erlanger, R.E. Heyman, K.D. O'Leary. "The honeymoon effect: does it exist and can it be predicted?" *Prev Sci.* 2015 May;16(4):550-9. doi: 10.1007/s11121-014-0480-4. PMID: 24643282.

Ma, Jiameng et al. "Effects of a workplace sit–stand desk intervention on health and productivity." *International Journal of Environmental Research and Public Health* 18.21 (2021): 11604.

Mahan, Brendan. "The Wall of Awful with Brendan Mahan." *Hacking Your ADHD*. Podcast, 19:30. https://www.hackingyouradhd.com/podcast/the-wall-of-awful-with-brendan-mahan.

Maki, P.M., E. Sundermann. (2009). "Hormone Therapy and Cognitive Function." *Hum Reprod Update*. https://doi.org//10.1093/humupd/dmp02.

Mayo Clinic. "Postpartum Depression." Accessed on November 1, 2023. https://www.mayoclinic.org/diseases-conditions/postpartum-depression/symptoms-causes/syc-20376617.

McMullen, Laura. "Impulse Buying: What It Is and How to Keep It in Check." NerdWallet. October 4, 2021. https://www.nerdwallet.com/article/finance/impulse-buying-definition.

MGH Center for Women's Mental Health. "New Study at the CWMH: Course of ADHD During Pregnancy and the Postpartum." August 16, 2017. https://womensmentalhealth.org/posts/course_adhd_pregnancy_postpartum/.

Mohebi, A., Berke, J.D. "Dopamine release drives motivation, independently from dopamine cell firing." *Neuropsychopharmacol.* 45, 220 (2020). https://doi.org/10.1038/s41386-019-0492-7.

Ptacek, R. et. al. "Clinical Implications of the Perception of Time in Attention Deficit Hyperactivity Disorder (ADHD): A Review." *Med Sci Monit.* 2019 May 26; 25:3918-3924. doi: 10.12659/MSM.914225. PMID: 31129679; PMCID: PMC6556068.

Puryear, D. (2012). *Your Life Can be Better: Using Strategies for Adult ADD/ADHD*. Mill City Press.

Rash, Joshua A., M. Kyle Matsuba, and Kenneth M. Prkachin. "Gratitude and well-being: Who benefits the most from a gratitude intervention?" *Applied Psychology: Health and Well-Being* 3.3 (2011): 350-369.

Santhi, N., A.S. Lazar, P.J. McCabe, J.C. Lo, J.A. Groeger, and D.J. Dijk. (2016). "Sex differences in the circadian regulation of sleep and waking cognition in humans."

Proceedings of the National Academy of Sciences of the United States of America, 113(19), E2730–E2739. https://pubmed.ncbi.nlm.nih.gov/27091961/.

Scarpelli, Serena, et al. "Advances in understanding the relationship between sleep and attention deficit-hyperactivity disorder (ADHD)." *Journal of Clinical Medicine* 8.10 (2019): 1737.

Sergeant, Joseph A. et al. "The top and the bottom of ADHD: a neuropsychological perspective." *Neuroscience & Biobehavioral Reviews* 27.7 (2003): 583-592.

Silananda, Sayadaw U. *The benefits of walking meditation*. Buddhist Publ. Society, 1995.

Silva, Alessandro P. et al. "Measurement of the effect of physical exercise on the concentration of individuals with ADHD." *PloS one* 10.3 (2015): e0122119.

Starck, Martina, Julia Grünwald, and Angelika A. Schlarb. "Occurrence of ADHD in parents of ADHD children in a clinical sample." *Neuropsychiatric Disease and Treatment* (2016): 581-588.

Wang, Y., J. Zhou, X. Gu, et al. The Effect of Self-Compassion on Impulse Buying: A Randomized Controlled Trial of an Online Self-Help Intervention." *Mindfulness* 14, 1542–1551 (2023). https://doi.org/10.1007/s12671-023-02139-y.

Villines, Zawn. "What is 'body doubling' for ADHD?" *Medical News Today*. August 24, 2023.
https://www.medicalnewstoday.com/articles/body-doubling-adhd.

Young, S., Adamo, N., Ásgeirsdóttir, B.B., et al. "Females with ADHD: An expert consensus statement taking a lifespan approach providing guidance for the identification and treatment of attention-deficit/ hyperactivity disorder in girls and women." *BMC Psychiatry* 20, 404 (2020). https://doi.org/10.1186/s12888-020-02707-9.

INDEX

imagination broadening, 36–37

"impression management," 30

impulse spending, 100–101, 105–108

impulsivity, 15

innovation, 36

insecure attachment, 32

internal clock, 141, 143

interruptions, controlling, 138–139

intimacy, 157–161

irritability, 15

J

Jiang, Jia, 28

jobs, 21, 23, 50–51, 57, 76. see also work life

K

knowledge constraint, 37

Kondo, Marie, 86

L

LePera, Nicole, 24

letting go of "stuff," 86

light, sleep and, 142–143

Ling, Lisa, 52–53

M

Mahan, Brendan, 172

masking, 29–31, 162–167

mastery, 41–42, 50

McCabe, Jessica, 99

mealtimes, 128–129

medications, 45, 115, 142

meditation
focus, 135–136
practice considerations, 136–137
unmasking, 166–167
walking, 137

melatonin, 142–143

menopause, 150–151

menstrual cycle, 150–152

mental stimulation, 45, 72–74

Methylphenidate, 115

Millburn, Joshua Fields, 86

mindfulness, 134–139

monophasic sleep, 140

mood swings, 15, 113

motivation, 72–74, 126, 149

N

National Birth Defects Prevention Study, 115

National Institutes of Health, 118, 153

nervous system dysregulation, 52, 170

neurodiversity, 21, 29, 30–31, 36, 51, 173

neurotypical, meaning of, 21

Nicodemus, Ryan, 86

"no," saying, 48

norepinephrine, 142, 150

note-taking, 138

novelty in relationships, 159–160

O

object permanence, 78

object retrieval, 78

OHIO acronym, 80

100-hour rule, 41–42

P

parenting
burnout, 120–126
generational ADHD, 127–131
postpartum adjustment, 116–119
pregnancy, 111–115

passion in relationships, 158–160

perfectionism, 42

perimenopause, 150

permission, asking for, 139

personality traits, 46–47

physical activity, 46, 52, 72–73, 114, 146–149

planning ability, 15

Pomodoro Technique, 43, 74

positive psychology, 123

postpartum adjustment, 116–119

pregnancy, 111–115

Price, Devon, 21

prioritization skills, 15

productivity, 41, 43

progesterone, 112, 150–151

puberty, 150

Puryear, Douglas, 78

ACKNOWLEDGMENTS

I would like to thank my clients who actively participated in creating this book. Your honesty and willingness to share your experiences to help other women with ADHD thrive is a beautiful testament to the community we all are. I would also like to thank my editor, Kim Suarez, at Zeitgeist/Penguin Random House and my developmental editor, Patty Consolazio, for consistently supporting all my ideas and iterations. You always encouraged whatever direction my creativity and passions took me and truly allowed me to embody what it means to "think outside the box" while writing this book.

I would also like to acknowledge the support of my family, who consistently gives me courage to explore my wide variety of passions and interests. When I come to you and say, "I have an idea" and the response is almost unanimously a loving smile and endless support, you unclip my wings and allow me to fly. This type of support, more than anything, is what I want for all the women reading this book.

Finally, I want to acknowledge you, the reader. To make monumental shifts in the way we think about ADHD in women demands that we explore new perspectives and challenge old ways of thinking. When we accept ADHD, not as a disorder but as a set of unique skills and adaptations, we are serving as pioneers forging a new path. Without this desire to learn and grow, we would never have books like this, and so for you, the reader, I am eternally grateful.

ABOUT THE AUTHOR

DR. AMELIA KELLEY is a trauma-informed therapist, author, podcaster, and researcher. Her specialties include art therapy, internal family systems (IFS), eye movement desensitization and reprocessing (EMDR), and brainspotting. She is also a certified meditation and yoga instructor. Her work focuses on women's issues, empowering survivors of abuse and relationship trauma, highly sensitive people, motivation, healthy living, and adult ADHD.

Dr. Kelley is currently a psychology professor at Yorkville University and a nationally recognized relationship expert. She is co-host of *The Sensitivity Doctors* podcast and has been featured on SiriusXM Doctor Radio's *The Psychiatry Show* as well as NPR's *The Measure of Everyday Life*. Her private practice is part of the Traumatic Stress Research Consortium at the Kinsey Institute. Dr. Kelley is the author of *Gaslighting Recovery for Women: The Complete Guide to Recognizing Manipulation and Achieving Freedom from Emotional Abuse* and co-author of *What I Wish I Knew: Surviving and Thriving After an Abusive Relationship*, and of *Surviving Suicidal Ideation: From Therapy to Spirituality and the Lived Experience*, and a contributing author for *Psychology Today* as well as the Highly Sensitive Refuge, the world's largest blog for HSPs. Her work has been featured in *Teen Vogue, Yahoo News, Life Hacker*, and *Insider*. You can find out more about her work at ameliakelley.com.

Hi there,

We hope you found *Powered by ADHD* helpful. If you have any questions or concerns about your book, or have received a damaged copy, please contact customerservice@penguinrandomhouse.com. We're here and happy to help.

Also, please consider writing a review on your favorite retailer's website to let others know what you thought of the book.

Sincerely,
The Zeitgeist Team